PRAISE FOR *YOGA TO SUPPORT IMMUNITY*

"This book is for anyone who wants to lovingly, persistently, and mindfully step forward into their best life. While *Yoga to Support Immunity* is certainly a powerful resource for wellness, recovery, and health, it is also a whole-life and spirit-awakening that supports seekers to shine the light of their awareness into the nooks and crannies of daily living. Melanie Salvatore-August irresistibly beckons you to make the practical real-life changes that will nourish your body and soul."

—Rachel Scott, MSc, MFA, E-RYT 500, YACEP, author, yoga teacher, and educational expert

"Melanie Salvatore-August offers us a widening view of what it means to be resilient and well by bolstering our immunity—physically, emotionally, mentally, and spiritually. Her program in *Yoga to Support Immunity* brings the ancient healing art of yoga to help us meet today's complex challenges by supporting our own innate healing powers and expanding our well-being."

—Jillian Pransky, author of *Deep Listening: A Healing Practice to Calm Your Body, Clear Your Mind, and Open Your Heart*

"At a time when  lth are needed more than ever, along te of Melanie Salvatore-August in h nity. With simple, step-by-step insi oward small, daily choices which improve immune function and cultivate whole body health. A brilliantly designed guide to vitality and resilience through yoga!"

—Darnell Cox, MA, RYT, holistic nutritionist and health coach

"*Yoga to Support Immunity* is a meditative guide to ease chronic stress, calm the nervous system, and heal the body. Melanie Salvatore-August offers a generous and grounded approach to yoga at its best—a steady, reliable reinforcement for holistic health and vitality, body and mind."

—Sarah Hays Coomer, NBC-HWC, NSCA-CPT, author of *The Habit Trip*, *Physical Disobedience*, and *Lightness of Body and Mind*

"A delightful guide for exploring the benefits of yoga as a path to being healthy, whole, and complete. Full of information in an easy-to-follow format, Melanie complied a program that is perfect for the individual to develop a practice on their own or in a group. I am happy to add this guide to the resources I recommend to my students and teachers."

—Jenni Maiwald Wendell, founder and creator of Just Be Yoga LLC and The Luminary Farm

"As physicians, we are deeply trained in the scientific method and critical analytical thinking as we approach patients and clinical situations. Practicing with Melanie Salvatore-August, I learned of deeper understandings in the realm of the experiential and intuitive yoga practice, a more subtle yet powerful approach to healing, but one that does not exclude our Western medical knowledge. In the pages of *Yoga to Support Immunity*, Melanie teaches a deep wisdom of the body and life's energies that we can each understand and use for our growth and well-being."

—Dr. Dale Poppert, MS, MD, FACEP

YOGA

TO SUPPORT IMMUNITY

YOGA

TO SUPPORT IMMUNITY

Mind, Body, Breathing Guide
to Whole Health

AUTHOR MELANIE SALVATORE-AUGUST

ARTIST SEBASTIAN ALAPPAT

yellow pear press

CORAL GABLES

Published by Yellow Pear Press, an imprint of Mango Publishing, a division of Mango Publishing Group, Inc.

Cover Design and Illustration: © Sebastian Alappat
Illustrations: © Sebastian Alappat
Art Direction: Morgane Leoni

For permission requests, please contact the publisher at:

Mango Publishing Group
2850 S Douglas Road, 2nd Floor
Coral Gables, FL 33134 USA
info@mango.bz

For special orders, quantity sales, course adoptions and corporate sales, please email the publisher at sales@mango.bz. For trade and wholesale sales, please contact Ingram Publisher Services at customer.service@ingramcontent.com or +1.800.509.4887.

Yoga to Support Immunity: Mind, Body, Breathing Guide to Whole Health

Library of Congress Cataloging-in-Publication number: 2021936163
ISBN: (print) 978-1-64250-572-6, (ebook) 978-1-64250-573-3
BISAC category code HEA025000—HEALTH & FITNESS / Yoga

Printed in the United States of America

Liability Statement: Always consult a physician before you begin a new exercise or breathing regime. The content in this book is to be of support only. It is not to replace medical supervision, advice, or prescriptions. There are inherent risks in any new regime, and you are fully responsible for your health and safety. The publisher and the author make no guarantees concerning the level of success you may experience by following the advice and strategies contained in this book, and you accept the risk that results will differ for each individual.

TO ALL OF MY TEACHERS, ESPECIALLY MOM, DAD,

RAFAEL, GIOVANNI, CASCIATO, AND ROMAN.

I AM FOREVER GRATEFUL FOR EVERY BIT OF YOU

AND OUR PRECIOUS TIME TOGETHER.

CONTENTS

PART I: CLARITY

PART II: DETOXIFICATION

PART III: INTEGRATION

FOREWORD

There are some people in this world whose presence expands your own sense of self. These are the people who meet you at the heart, who validate you, who speak with honesty and compassion, and who stand firmly yet humbly in their own light. Melanie Salvatore-August is one of these people. She has always been a truly radiant being.

I first met Melanie when she was the manager of Yoga Works in NYC. These were in my early years of teaching, before my husband and I opened the ISHTA Yoga studio in 2008. Mel and I would often exchange words between my classes. They were kind words that always left me with a sense of lightness, whether it was around the topic of yoga anatomy or what to order for lunch. She conveyed a sense of confidence that was comforting and nonintimidating. I knew she lived a life of meaning, and I admired it deeply.

Now, over fifteen years later, I reflect on my relationship with Melanie as a sort of sisterhood from afar. Although we currently live on opposite sides of the country, there is an unspoken camaraderie between us that is genuine and unique, especially for women who are in the same industry. As fellow lululemon ambassadors, Melanie and I have always shared a common sense of purpose in the work we do as yoga teachers. She developed her own organization, Fierce Kindness, through which she raised awareness of the harmful effects of bullying that pervades our culture. I served on the board of Exhale to Inhale, a nonprofit organization that provides the healing powers of yoga to survivors of domestic violence and sexual assault. Regardless of where we were or what we were embarking on, we cheered each other on from the sidelines. Even if I questioned my own place in the world, Melanie's generosity of spirit reminded me how much I mattered. I know that that generosity is a gift she shares with everyone she comes in contact with.

When Melanie approached me about doing a benefit class for Exhale to Inhale in 2015, her vision was to bring together female teachers for a common cause, accompanied by live music. We co-taught one of the most magical classes I have ever offered, alongside Elena Brower. Witnessing Melanie in her purpose of sharing and elevating others through yoga was an inspiration to me.

Melanie is a true leader. She is a mother, a wife, a teacher, and an author. She is a yogini. In this age of information, there are so many different permutations of what yoga is. Those who truly live it are few and far between. I have had the great honor of working with luminaries such as Deepak Chopra, Gabby Bernstein, and Seane Corn, all of whom have mastered that art. I have also been blessed to learn daily from my husband, yoga master Alan Finger. Living a modern life based on spiritual concepts might seem like a contradiction, but I believe it is necessary for our sustainability. Melanie not only embodies the wisdom of yoga, she disseminates it with friendliness and ease.

In the ancient text, the *Bhagavad Gita,* yoga is referred to as "a journey of the self, through the self, to the self." At a time in our world when we are experiencing a social, economic, and health crisis unlike anything we have experienced in our lifetime, yoga is no longer a luxury. It is a necessity. The world is desperate for true healing, and the only way it will happen is if we learn how to heal ourselves. The practices that Melanie has unearthed in this book are profound because they are inherent within each one of us. We don't need to download an app or order any special equipment to access them. We simply need to be reminded of our own innate power as a member of the human species.

The origin of the word *health* is related to the word "whole," or a thing that is complete in itself.[1] When we integrate all aspects of our being, we are in a state of health. Our modern Western society often mistakes yoga for a physical exercise or a belief system, when actually it is a science of becoming whole. To dismiss the yogic benefits of breath, meditation, mantra, and visualization is like celebrating only one color of the rainbow. What this book offers is the entire spectrum of the yoga practice. It is targeted, practical, authentic, and poetic all at the same time.

We are on the threshold of a new era, where virtues such as inclusivity, justice, empathy, and awareness are all being called upon for our global healing. However,

---

1   https://www.ncbi.nlm.nih.gov/pmc/articles/PMC3917469/

we cannot find those virtues "out there" if we cannot find them in here. *Yoga to Support Immunity* is a practical guide to unlocking the seeds of potential that are latent within each one of us. Regardless of your background, creed, or political preference, you deserve to feel whole. May this book serve to create transformation on an individual level so that we realize true peace and harmony as a collective.

—SARAH PLATT FINGER
February 8, 2021
Cofounder, ISHTA Yoga

INTRODUCTION

YOGA IS AN EXPERIENCE OF WHOLE-BEING HARMONY

The Sanskrit word *yoga* translates to yoke or unify. Also synonymous with physical exercise, the *asanas* or yoga poses are utilized to bring health, flexibility and focus. Postural practices can bring about an experience of yoga. Yet it is only one of the ways to experience the state of yoga or unification of the whole self.

The earliest philosophy and practices to invoke yoga came out of the Indus Valley, an area which roughly spans from northeast Afghanistan to northwest India, over five thousand years ago. They were centered around directing the mind and breathing to create a realization of wholeness and present-state absorption, or yoga. The physical asanas or poses we know now, developed over the last five hundred years, or so are relatively new in the lineage of a yoga practice. The postural yoga is Hatha Yoga; there are also Karma Yoga, the yoga of selfless service; Bhakti Yoga, the yoga of devotion and spirit; Jnana Yoga, the yoga of wisdom and self-realization; and Raja Yoga, the yoga of dissolving mental barriers. We utilize all of the forms of yoga for whole health in this book.

For me, yoga is a way of living, a guiding sense of loving wholeness that directs my thoughts, actions, and my days into joyful presence. I have been studying and practicing various aspects of yoga since I was an adolescent in the eighties, and I have been teaching the practice full-time since 2006. Over the last fifteen years, I have taught hundreds of people and had the honor of sharing and supporting their healing journey of yoga. I am not a doctor, nor do I consider myself a master—I'm a busy mother of three, a dedicated practitioner, and a regular person who has utilized yoga to help heal herself and support many others. The tools I share are timeless, scientifically supported, and delivered in a practical way, so that a busy, earnest person can integrate them.

IMMUNITY IS RESILIENCE AGAINST DISEASE

Immunity is when we have protection, resilience, and endurance to withstand an attack and continue to thrive. In our physiology, it is the ability to fight viruses, recalibrate and balance the microbiome, and assimilate important nutrients, as well as detoxify from environmental predators and pollutants. Mentally and emotionally, it is our ability to discern what we need or don't need and to create peace within our everyday life.

YOGA CREATES RESILIENCE AND DIRECTLY SUPPORTS IMMUNE FUNCTION

When we are experiencing a state of wholeness or yoga, our nervous system moves into the parasympathetic response, or rest/digest state. This state of rest/digest supports the longevity functions of digestion, hormone balance, and immunity. There are numerous tools to access a state of yoga supporting the immune system, and I share many of these throughout this book.

Whole health immunity is based on the quality of our exercise, breathing, stress levels, sleep, relationships, diet, and genetics. It is also based on what we repeatedly do each day or our habits. This book of yoga practices addresses all of these areas except diet, relationships, and genetics. Yet I have found that, when aligned in the above areas, we naturally begin to choose more nourishing foods, as well as healthier relationships, to support our life, and that supports us more gracefully in handling the cards we have been dealt, meaning our genetics.

STEADINESS IS THE GATEWAY TO YOGA AND IMMUNITY

The state of yoga comes from systemic harmony and the ability to sit still without physical or mental discomfort. We do asanas (poses) so the body is flexible, strong, and pain-free to remain in a quiet state for an extended period of time.

Asanas clear inflammation and dis-ease from the body. The body and mind work together. If the mind is agitated, the body will have difficulty being still. If the body is in pain, the mind will be agitated. Like waves on a lake, the water will be disturbed and murky without visibility to the bottom. When our mind and body are quiet, just as the still lake water is clear, we can see all the way into the depths of our experience. When aspects of us are disjointed, we experience confusion, anxiety, depression, illness, and disease.

BREATHING IS THE BRIDGE BETWEEN THE BODY AND THE MIND

Our breath is a direct gateway to our power and whole-being health. The higher mind and consciousness (which you may call essential self, soul, or spirit) is the witness; the breath carries the information of the body's and mind's physical experience back to the self. The breath and mind/body are reciprocal. When the breath is smooth and long, the body and mind (where emotions are held) are at peace. When the breath is short and jagged, the body and mind (emotions) are disturbed. The quality of our breath is the most important factor in whole health and is one of the main areas of focus in this book.

YOGA CREATES WHOLE-BEING HARMONY AND FIGHTS DISEASE

The practices of yoga bring the right and left hands together in harmony (versus one hand cleaning while the other hand creates a mess). When our heart is telling us one thing, our mind is pulling us in the opposite direction, and the body has completely revolted; we suffer and experience dis-ease.

The journey of yoga and whole health is uniquely personal. For this reason, we start with the foundation of inquiries to create personal clarity on what you are repeatedly desiring, thinking, feeling, and doing as a source of energy and power. When we do practices based on this personal clarity, they are amplified and more effective.

Spinal health, circulation, digestion, elimination, inflammation reduction, and hormone balance are our main focus areas for the asanas to support immune function. We will breathe deeply through the nose, increasing production of nitric oxide, which is a health booster, and de-stress our nervous system for resilience and healing. Utilizing the expansive muscles of the breath, we will learn to reset the nervous system out of a chronic stress response and rewire our system for deep calm and resilience. We will explore daily habits to eliminate those that drain us and cultivate those that energize us, creating an easy consistency.

There is no magic pill or one-time effort. Immunity support and whole health are based on small, daily choices that create a resilient vitality over time. Utilizing the yogic principles of *abhyasa* and *vairagya*, or the balanced recipe of consistency and nonattachment, the accumulative effects can be life-changing. With this book, create daily habits that you engage in with a sense of contentment and ease. Keep going and don't give up, while cultivating an "oh well" attitude to imperfections. Release the goal or outcome while enjoying the journey of the practice. The flow of the journey will be just right for you and will be *your yoga*.

START WHERE YOU ARE, USE WHAT YOU HAVE, AND HELPFUL WAYS TO USE THIS BOOK

These real healing practices are for real people. You have everything you need to start this journey and create the next level of vitality. It only takes one small shift in awareness to create a big healing change. Whether it is a shift in how you breathe, how you move, or how you perceive your life, there will be benefit. It doesn't matter if you have lots of experience with these healing practices or none; just take a deep breath, accept whatever gifts or challenges feel present, and keep going. The only thing that is needed is curiosity and a desire to be supported right now. Don't worry about tomorrow and don't get stuck in the past—just steadily keep going in the present, as the present moment is truly all we have and where the healing occurs.

These practices are meant to be layered and serve as entry points for you to be supported in whatever healing focus you choose. The healing wisdom is inside you, and this book is to support you to listen more deeply and to offer reminders of areas you may have forgotten. Read and practice along with the book in a linear manner, which I recommend especially if you are new to yoga—or, if you are already quite experienced with the practice, start with the area of greatest support. I also recommend, if possible, that you follow along with the audio recording of this book so you can be led in real time when practicing. If for whatever reason that is not possible, consider downloading the individual tutorials for the main practices in this book from my website melaniesalvatoreaugust.com.

My whole life has led me to this moment, and it is an honor to share these tools with you. I have learned along the way that nothing is wasted, no time, experience, or effort. It is all a perfect strand of this beautiful tapestry of awakening to love and wholeness.

Fear drains us of our vitality, and love (both self-love and universal love) will fuel our immunity and whole health. I support you in choosing love, compassion, and patience when practicing these tools and allowing the practice to gently bless you one breath at a time. There is unbound potential within this practice to bring us to whole-being harmony or yoga; they have transformed my health and life, and I hope they bless yours as well.

HOW THIS BOOK WORKS

There are three main sections (Parts I, II, and III), each containing one practical conceptual chapter with inquiries for self-study to support you getting clearer on what you need and why, other chapters with *asanas* (physical postures) and *pranayamas* (breathing exercises and meditations), and one chapter with practice sequences to help you move into action. Both the movement and the breathing chapters include helpful images, step by step how-to instructions, detailed immunity benefits, effects, and essential tidbits to consider for each exercise to boost enthusiasm, because when we understand the why, the what becomes much easier.

The breathing section can also include specific *kriyas* or cleansing techniques, a *mudra* or energy seal, and focused awareness meditation to lead you into deep healing calm. The sequence chapters also contain Three-Minute and Eight-Minute Sequences for effective movement and breathing sessions that are easy to incorporate into your daily life. Chapter 12, the final sequence chapter, includes longer practice sequences focused on mild illness support, gentle illness recovery, and additional, vigorous practices focused on creating balance, strength and vitality. Each sequence section also includes a resource of a kriya/pranayama practice to support the deeper mind and body practice. This gives you a wide range of meal choices for whatever the needs of the day and life call for.

Each part closes with a summary section highlighting the essential takeaway and an "Only one thing? Do this" tip to give you another entry point if you feel you are low on time.

The organization of the tools is inspired by the five winds of *prana* or life force energy. In the yogic and Ayurvedic systems, the *Pancha Vayus*, or five pranic winds, govern the functions of our body. The Five Pranas break down to the *prana* or energy of nourishment, *prana-vayu*; the prana of *apana*, or detoxification and moving out byproduct; the prana of assimilation or focus, utilizing or homing in on what is nourishing, which is called *samana*; *udana*, the prana of outward movement; and finally *vyana*, the prana of circulation and integration of the other four pranic winds for whole health radiance.

I share with you here the multidimensional exploration of how to create whole health by balancing these flows of energy. What are you taking in? How are you eliminating what is no longer needed? What are you actually absorbing and integrating that makes a difference? When these five pranic *vayus* are balanced, we are resilient and radiant with whole health, and our immunity is strong.

Each practice here is shared to inspire you to create your own healing yoga practice that supports you, whether in mild illness, in gentle recovery, or in maintaining already vibrant health. That said, please be advised that these practices are not to replace important professional care for serious illness, injury, or trauma. Any acute disease, or physical or mental health issues are to be aided with supervised, expert care; the tools in this book, although helpful, are meant for the average healthy person to create daily whole health practices based in the lineage of yoga, and are reinforced by science.

I hope that you integrate these simple, yet potent, tools into your life. When you are in need of grounding, a boost in self-care, inspiration, and inner quiet, I hope that just the right page opens to you and it supports your own inner listening to guide you back to peace and whole health.

Healing comes from within. We have the power to heal ourselves—no one else can do it for us; it is truly an inside job. Yes, of course, our healing process can either be supported or undermined by outside forces, yet the true aspect of healing is up to our own body, connected to our deeper essential consciousness, being aligned within our daily actions.

Getting intentional with our actions is one of most the powerful tools for immunity and resilience, as it focuses our reticular activating system, an important nerve command center in the brain. As above as it is below. We see the vibrant canopy of the oak tree, yet it is the intricate expansive root system underneath that holds it up. The canopy will be your health and wellness, and these intentional practices will help you create the strong root system below.

Focus on the practice, not the product or performance. Trust and enjoy the process, releasing any struggle or push for outcome. Align your body and mind with this flow of yoga, and you will be naturally potent, radiant, and resilient.

PREPARATION FOR YOUR YOGA PRACTICE

Our success is supported in our preparation. These simple considerations in preparation for the practice will help make doing the practice easier. Getting started can be the hardest part, so whatever can make that first step easier will benefit us. After you get going, the rest will fall into place.

If possible, practice on an empty stomach, at least two hours after a meal. Avoid drinking water during a practice, and hydrate well before and after. Cultivate *saucha* or cleanliness in each step of your practice: come to practice clean, practice in a clean environment, and guide your thoughts to supportive positivity.

The number of times you practice will affect the success of your experience. The more you can repeat the mind-body practices in this book, the more chance they will take effect and become ingrained in your automatic patterns of self-care. We want the introspection, the moving of the body, the breathing to reset your nervous system, and the breathing peacefully each day all to become a way of life.

HOW TO SET YOURSELF UP FOR SUCCESS

Get a yoga journal or notebook to record your musings from the inquiries in this book. There are many moments of *svadhyaya* or self-study included here, and free-writing your responses will be helpful in bringing information from the recesses of the mind forward in your awareness. Log your experiences with the practices as they come up. Consider keeping the journal where you practice for brief after-practice downloads.

Designate a small clean area for your practice—if possible, a location where there are fewer distractions, no other people, and where you have access to a wall is ideal. Make sure it is tidy and intentional so that, when you step into the space, you have an immediate recall of the intention for healing and your system moves into that response just by being there.

Keep whatever yoga support props you use in view and at the ready. When you see your mat, yoga blocks, journal with pen, favorite yoga blanket, or meditation shawl, you will immediately be reminded to practice and desire to do so.

You do not need any props. That said, props help the body hold alignment and can help make the postures safer, as they may stop the body from slipping or falling over. I share my favorite props and how to get them in the resources section at the end of this book.

Consider having:

- a natural rubber yoga mat
- two firm foam yoga blocks or two sturdy large books
- a strap or a long old tie
- two yoga blankets or two large firm bath towels
- an eye mask or pillow or a small towel or rolled-up black T-shirt can do the trick as well

Write down your commitment to practicing in your calendar or on your to-do list.

Be as specific as you can, for example: *"On Monday, at 7:15 a.m., right after I wake up, before I make my coffee, I will do three yoga poses and one breathing practice and sit for one minute in a quiet state."* The more specific you can be as to what and when, the more likely the outcome will be.

After practice, log that you did it to support the sense of accomplishment.

Prep the activity earlier in the day or the night before. Planning to practice right after you wake up? Roll out your mat, and place your journal and pen on the mat in preparation. Before walking away, see yourself practicing tomorrow in your mind's eye. Do an inner mini-rehearsal (even one second of seeing yourself do it will plant the seed of success) before you walk away.

Reset the space for the next time. (This one is a game-changer for me personally.) As you are already in the flow, resetting the space will take a fraction of the time that it will later on, cold. For example, after my practice, I gather my blocks, refold my blankets, roll my strap, and place them all, neatly stacked, to the side, waiting for the next day. I tidy any lint or debris and fully reset the space to be ready. I take a second to pause and see myself there the next day, practicing in my mind's eye as an intention-setting mini-rehearsal.

Choose the Three-Minute Essential Daily Sequence, or a couple of simple asanas, to practice in the "must use" areas, like the bathroom or the kitchen, consistently. These are places you go daily and throughout the day, which are a must. You don't have to think about going there; you will do it automatically. As long as there is no water on the floor or other dangers, these are great locations to add a desired practice on top of routine activities. Washing your hands at the sink? Finish drying hands and add a couple of Full Complete Breaths, a standing Sun Stretch, and a simple Lunge position on both legs before you walk out. As you do the poses, remember to breathe deeply through the nose and remember your intentions to heal and get stronger. The more you practice, the greater the accumulative effects. Practice in your intentional location, as well as everywhere else, throughout your day.

Do a mental rehearsal. Right now, with me. If it is safe to do so, close your eyes and, with your inner vision, see yourself happily doing the above preparations and the yoga practices. See yourself breathing deeply and feeling clear, hopeful, and strong. Seeing it sets the intention and places the sequence into your brain, as well as programming the RAS, or reticular activating system, which is a part of the brain that helps us see opportunities to access support.

Preparation is helpful, yet the imperfect doing is the key. Just do the practice imperfectly. To keep failing forward is the true key to success. The doing gives us the experience of yoga or whole-being harmony. Every time we practice, we learn and grow.

It is the sheer action that will create whole health and immunity. Let's not hesitate or wait to do the practice; let's start doing it right now.

PART I

CLARITY

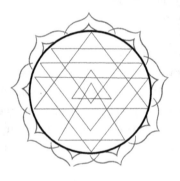

CHAPTER 1

AWARENESS AND ALIGNMENT

It only takes one small shift in awareness to create a big healing change.

What we think, how we feel, and what we do have significant impact on our immunity and whole health. It is the small things we do consistently that have the greatest impact on our life. What we value directly affects how we move and take care of our bodies. Therefore, the first area of foundational exploration is our personal thought processes and then how that translates into physical action. We will peer into ourselves to get clarity on what we want and need, observing our habitual patterns and then applying new, helpful ones based on science and yogic sense.

Clarity on what is needed, as well as where the challenges lie, are key for this successful journey. Clarity on what you want to cultivate and what you need to clear creates a synergy with positive results.

For me, self-study is the most important and difficult frontier. It seems easy to see someone else clearly, yet it is harder to see and be honest with ourselves. Often harmful habits are fulfilling some deeper need and are therefore difficult, or even on the surface undesirable, to get rid of. Please don't make me get real on the fact that my caffeine-packed extra-large cup of coffee is not to my benefit; I am just not ready to face it! Yoga offers step by step support for shifting unhelpful habits and integrating new helpful ones.

Our yoga practice will fortify *samskaras* (SAHM-ska-rahs), or habits for transformation, cultivated by *sankalpa*s (SAHN-kahl-pahs), seeds of heart intention. We want to plant a clear heart intention into our conscious mind so it will root into our subconscious and change the way we process on a neurological and cellular level.

To prevent our mind from becoming overloaded by the mass of daily tasks and choices, much of our brain processing is automatic and does not utilize the conscious mind. This is one of the reasons it may be hard to get to the root of our habits and why this self-study approach can be helpful. A relaxed, curious, and contented approach to this process will support you in a receptive space and help open the window into the subconscious mind. Struggle begets struggle, so focus on what feels doable today or this week. Consider not overhauling everything all at once and addressing the most accessible tasks first. The success momentum will affirm you forward. Necessity will be the mother of *intervention*, so trust the timing of when you will address what area. If it is an area of necessity that feels very challenging, consider reaching out to a professional for additional support.

This section, Part I, will focus on adding in positive, immediately actionable habits. In Part II, Detoxification, we will explore how to shift out of harmful habits, and Part III will support us in creating a playground of practice to focus on what is working, free ourselves for resistance, and integrate healing, creating a tipping point effect for big change.

The physical body is the most tangible place for us to begin, and getting clear on our why will energize us into the asanas (AH-sa-nahs), or poses, to exercise the body. It's better to move the body for a short time every day then to exercise for a couple of hours once a week. Our strategy is to weave the movement of the body into the everyday, just like brushing teeth and, *ahem*, making coffee. This is the way to establish consistency, which will have an accumulative effect that supports healing change.

Movement of the body and yoga poses do not have to be complex or intimidating. In fact, most often the simplest postures are the best, as they carry less risk from injury. We look at what we are gaining, and then look at where we are at risk to lose, and it creates a simple cost analysis for us. Keep the posture basic, and there is lots to gain and little to lose. When we practice the more complex poses, headstand for example, the risk of injury to the neck can outweigh the benefits, and we can experience similar benefits with a different, safer posture. Neck, shoulders, lower back, and knees are "expensive" injuries, so proceed with caution on more complex postures. Stick with what is immediately accessible for you that can be practiced while remaining steady and relaxed. If those more complex postures are a burning desire for you, consider asking why that is, what is at the root of the desire, and whether it supports whole health. If it does, then find a qualified yoga teacher in your area and begin studying with them so they can support you step by step, safely, in and out of the posture.

Spinal movement is key in our physical health. Extension of the spine (as in a good stretch within a gentle back bend), flexion (like fetal position), lateral flexion and extension (side stretching), and gentle rotation in the upper middle spine, practiced daily, will aid disc and joint health, circulation, and inflammation reduction.

We want to increase circulation and decrease inflammation. Inflammation is a part of our body's defense system and is a chemical reaction to invaders or injury. Acute inflammation is shorter-lived and often a response to a specific injury or illness. Chronic inflammation can be systemic, low-grade, and continue for years. Studies have shown that contributors to chronic inflammation include lack of exercise, irritating foods, stress, lack of sleep, obesity, low-grade chronic infection, and it can simply come with aging.

When we sit or don't move for long periods of time, we get stiff. That stiffness is caused by lack of movement of blood, lymphatic and synovial fluids, which become stagnated. That stagnation creates swelling and inflammation. A way for us to stave off chronic stiffness is to gently move the spine in all directions every day, as well as throughout the day.

Our job is to make spinal movement our daily habit.

Spinal movements could easily be incorporated while standing in your bathroom each morning or sitting at your desk each afternoon—any place or time you could consistently do something that would lend to the practice.

Spinal movements also stimulate the internal organs supporting many key players in our immune system, such as the diaphragm, lungs, heart, intestines, liver, and the endocrine and lymphatic systems. The poses we will be practicing will move our spine in all directions and aid this essential healing movement through the whole body.

When we create spinal movement, stimulate circulation, and expand the breath, we also stimulate the vagus nerve, a special player in supporting whole health. The vagus nerve (like the word vagabond) is a wandering traveler that runs from the brain stem through the throat down to the colon. It is the longest cranial nerve, and its main function is to activate the parasympathetic nervous system response, which I will refer to here as the rest/digest response. Its job is to calm us down and to support our longevity functions of digestion, hormone balance, and immunity. Our yoga poses and breathing practices work directly with the vagus nerve to support our immune system.

The *Bhagavad Gita*, one of the seminal texts of yoga, in Chapter 2 at line fifty, states, "Yoga is skill in action." Ultimately it is a practice of doing: doing intentionally, with awareness. That is perfect for us, here in modern life, as we are a bunch of doers and like to do all over the place. With a refined clarity, let us look at what we are already doing to see what is working, and what is *not* working, and identify our daily focus so as to redirect that focus to what will give us the greatest healing impact. Remember, it is what we repeatedly do that has the greatest impact on our whole health.

"Yoga is the quieting of the mind," states the second sutra, in the first chapter of the key wisdom text, the *Yoga Sutras of Patanjali*. Yoga is experienced when we quiet the inner dialogue to witness our true self. When we are connected to that capital-T Truth of who we are, the witness consciousness or essential self, beyond the constantly changing circumstances of life, our experience expands, and we tap into a larger view of possibility. What is true self? As defined by Samkhya Yoga and Patanjali's *Sutras*, the true self is the *purusha* (pooh-ROO-shah) or nonchanging being, witnessing the changeable aspects of the self, called prakriti (PRAH-kree-tee). When we forget or are ignorant of the fact that we are more than our constantly changing circumstances of thoughts, emotions, body, and relationships, we suffer. When we drop into the awareness, remembering or self-actualizing that we are the witness or essential self, we create an expansive resilience and a joyful life.

Yoga is not a religion; it is a practice and a philosophy of living. To give context for the practices utilized in this book, it is helpful to look at the practice as defined by the Eight Limbs in the *Yoga Sutras of Patanjali*. Through these eight limbs of yoga, we can create an experience of whole-being harmony, and through that harmony, we support our immune function.

Each limb builds on the next with intentional sequence, like steps of a staircase. The outer and inward observances and self-study prepare us for the *asanas* (AH-sah-na) or postural practice. The asanas prepare us for the healing work of the *pranayamas (PRAH-na-YAH-mahs)*. The pranayamas shift our nervous system and brain waves to help us draw into quiet and create inner focus. Focus and concentration lead us into a healing meditative state, connecting us to feeling of absorption or stillness called *samadhi* (sah-MAH-dee). If there is a yoga goal, that goal would be the deep nourishing quiet of *samadhi*, or total absorption, which brings us back to our essential self.

The real yoga is personal to you and your unique experience of wholeness. The experience of wholeness calms the nervous system and harmonizes the mind and body. A harmonized mind and body are more resilient and radiant with whole health immunity.

The mind, body, and breathing tools of the eight limbs of yoga support immunity, and they are as follows.

THE EIGHT LIMBS OF YOGA

- *Yama* (YAH-mah), outward observances (connecting with others)
  - *Ahimsa* (ah-HEEM-sah): non-violence
  - *Satya* (SAH-tyah): truthfulness
  - *Asteya* (ah-STAY-ya): non-stealing
  - *Brahmacharya* (BRAH-mah-CHAR-ee-ya): moderation
  - *Aparigraha* (a-PAIR-i-GRAH-ha): non-hoarding
- *Niyamas* (nee-YAH-mahs): Inward observances (connection with self)
  - *Saucha* (SOU-cha): cleanliness
  - *Santosha* (SAHN-to-sha): contentment
  - *Tapas* (tah-PAHS): heat or challenge for growth
  - *Svadhyaya* (SVAH-adyaa-ya): self-study
  - *Ishvara Pranidhana* (EESH-vahr-ah PRAH-nee-dah-nah): surrender
- *Asana* (AH-sah-na): physical postures (direct translation is "seat")
- *Pranayama* (PRAH-na-YAH-mah): breathing to direct prana (life force energy)
- *Pratyahara* (PRAH-tee-AH-hah-ra): drawing in of the outward senses into inner awareness
- *Dharana* (dhar-ah-nah): concentration
- *Dhyana* (DEE-yah-nah): prolonged concentration or meditation
- *Samadhi* (sah-MAH-dee): absorption into stillness

In this book, we will touch on all aspects of the eight limbs, yet do our deepest exploration with the self-study, physical postures, breathing exercises, and concentration/meditations. I hope it brings you to a sweet state of harmony and experience of wholeness.

PHYSICAL POSTURES

Postures are meant to be practiced in a progressive strength and relaxation building way. Not every pose is for every body, plus some poses are better practiced early in the day and others at night. Listen to your body in this exploration. Don't push or overpower the body with the desire to achieve what is in the picture or what is described. Practice gently, breath by breath and step by step, to be sensitive to the body's cues of what is enough or too much.

If you feel pain, that is a cue to stop.

Vinyasa krama (vin-YAH-sah krah-ma), which you may be familiar with as vinyasa yoga or flow yoga, is directly translated as "to place in a special way, step by step," or breath by breath. The "special way" is the way that is sustainable for you, and creating a harmony of balanced effort that is experienced through feeling steady yet spacious in each breath and in each pose.

Do postures to strengthen and release tension from the body, and as an exploration ground for the deeper intention work of self-study.

Observe your patterns.

How you do things here is a view into how you may do things in your life. When or where you force is an important space of observation. When do you cultivate struggle, making something harder than it needs to be? Observe when you avoid or bypass to get further ahead in some way. Just notice and breathe to access your own compassion for yourself. This is a friendly compassionate practice, and it starts with how you talk to and treat yourself.

BREATHING EXERCISES TO DIRECT LIFE FORCE

When the body hurts, or has a lot of sensation, it is difficult to focus on the breathing, and even more difficult to calm the mind to concentrate; that is why we generally start with the asanas to get the body feeling stable. Then we go into the breath.

The breath is the bridge between the physical body, the nervous system, and the mind. Our breath keeps us alive as well as signaling the brain/nervous system to let us know if we are safe or if we are in danger. When we are safe, the breath will move into full and smooth cadence, and when we perceive danger the breath will become shallow and fast.

Breathing is an automatic process and will happen when we have our attention on it or not. It is also a life-giving process that we can consciously shift and direct. Different breathing exercises can have different effects and, just like asanas, certain breathing patterns are best in the early hours of the day and others before bedtime. We will learn breathing to calm, heal, cool the mind/body, and heat and energize the mind/body, as well as detox.

CREATING CLARITY IS THE FOUNDATION OF POSTURES, BREATHING, AND MEDITATION

Through yoga, we create clarity through the three Ss: *svadhyaya* (SVAH-dee-yah-yah), which is self-study, *samskara* (sam-SKAH-rah), habits, patterns, and mental impressions, and *sankalpa* (san-KAHL-pah), our heart intention.

Self-study is the foundation of our yoga practice. You are the vehicle for this universal harmony and connection. Your journey starts with you and depends on what you think, feel, and do, all the time. Study your habitual patterns and discover how their accumulation creates your daily experience. With clarity on what is important for you, choose your actions in the world inspired by intention to create potency.

KNOW YOURSELF

What is essentially important to you? What is your desire for your life? Why have you chosen this book, this time, this body for this life, and what is the deep driving force or desire within you?

These life-changing inquiries are worthy of your time, patience, and attention. Where your attention goes, your prana or life force will follow, so invest your attention in exploring your why.

Your attention is your currency—use it wisely and, when you find that you are wasting it on something you don't want or that is draining you, shift it to what you do want and to areas of life that will help you to experience your heart's desires.

THE YOGA PRACTICE CREATES THE POWER TO PAUSE, FEEL, AND CHOOSE

In our yoga practice, we have the perfect contained space to observe how we react and respond to life. We have an arena to train ourselves to be sensitive to our inner cues, question our deeper why, and intentionally choose how we create our response. It is not the yogi pushup *chaturanga* that makes it the ultimate power practice; it is the power to pause, feel, and choose for our personal health and expansion.

THE WHY AFFECTS THE HOW, AND THE HOW CHANGES EVERYTHING

It can be difficult to get clarity on our why and then to get a hold of our how. That is why self-study is essential to this process. Use the guided self-inquiries to help focus in on what you need and how to create it. Full disclosure, I do a similar inventory on myself on a regular basis and am always fascinated by how, even though it may have only been a month's passing, I have changed, or there is something else revealed to me by taking a compassionate deeper look.

CREATING CLARITY ON THE BIGGER VIEW

Consider writing in a journal or notebook. Get settled into a peaceful spot for introspection and take some time to breathe into and explore these inquiries.

- What is the most important or essential thing to you right now?
- What is important or essential to you long-term for the bigger picture?
- What is your main objective for your life?
- What is your main objective for this yoga practice?
- How can you give more love in all aspects of your life and be more of service in the world?
- Do any of the above answers align or overlap? If so, how and where?
- What is *in the way* of you living what is essential to you, or the main obstacles?
- Summarize your answers into a few words as a seed of intentions in your life.

KNOW YOUR HABITS AND TENDENCIES

- In what ways do you take good care of yourself?
- In what ways do you harm yourself (*intentionally or unintentionally*)?
- Make a list of the things you do every day and, beside each, note whether you think the activity supports your health or detracts from it, as harmful, helpful, or neutral.

Examples:

Brush teeth	*Helpful!*
Go into the kitchen	*Neutral*
Check my phone	*Depends...maybe more harmful?*
Walk the dog	*Helpful*

- Where and when do you experience the most stress in your life?
- What would you like to do less of? What would you like to do more of?

- Would you categorize yourself as someone who pushes or as someone who is more passive?
- When do you push?
- When are you passive?

KNOW YOUR BODY

- What hurts in your body?
- What parts of your body are stiff? Strong? Flexible?
- What position does your body utilize most often? (sitting, standing, reclined)
- How do these positions help or harm you?
- How does this cause the body repetitive stress?
- How do you usually sit?
    Examples: Left foot tucked under hip or both feet on the floor, both sides of my body even and upright.

- How do you usually stand?
    Examples: Left leg and foot turned out, weight into right hip or both feet hip-width, parallel to each other, and upright.

- How do you usually lie down or sleep?
    Examples: On my back or curled onto left side with a pillow between thighs.

- What kind of shoes do you wear, and how many hours a day do you wear them?
- Do your shoes have a significant heel, higher than an inch?
- How do you think your shoes may affect the health of your feet, knees, and spine?

ARE YOU READY FOR THE LIFE-CHANGING PRACTICE OF YOGA?

This may seem like a strange question to pose at the end of these practical inquiries, yet it is possibly the most important one to ask. All the information, research, and discussions of benefits in the world will not be effective if we are not willing and ready to heal. I am hoping that, since you picked up this book, the answer is yes.

The process of self-inquiry, pausing to feel and making a conscious choice instead of a habitual, unconscious choice, creates whole health. There is joy in this path. There is an energy of delight created when the heart, the mind, and the body work together in skilled doing. Yoga is experienced in the now-present moment. Now is the time of yoga, and being ready is a part of the initiation of the practice. Trust the process that, if you have gotten this far, even if you feel a sense of slight nervousness or stirring discomfort, you are ready. Consider creating forward energy movement by declaring out loud or in writing:

I AM READY.

I AM READY FOR YOGA.

I AM READY FOR HEALING AND WHOLE-BEING HEALTH.

I trust the process, and I am excited for you to go deeper into the process of creating your whole-being harmony.

Keep these journal inquiry responses for future explorations. Let's get moving into the postures and where we will continue to build on this whole health transformation.

CHAPTER 2

ASANA FOR CLARITY

Our yoga asanas, or poses, are physical exercises that strengthen the body and decrease inflammation while increasing circulation throughout the body. This chapter focuses on spinal health, foundational habit patterns, and how to integrate doing postures with intention to stabilize the body and mind to begin the activation of the healing rest/digest response.

In this chapter, we will explore how to stabilize the spine, align the joints, strengthen the base of the core, and use the body as the anchor to steady the mind. Within our practice, we have the opportunity to further optimize the mind by activating the intentions with each posture, creating embodiment or tangible experience of our inner life. We will practice this embodiment, weaving mind, body, and breathing together intentionally here as the foundations of our healing practice. If the mind and present consciousness is not anchored into the postures, it creates an appliance without electricity and undermines the potency of the practice. This is why we start repeatedly with intention of the mind, then the body and beyond. Please kindly note that when we practice *mindlessly*, we create opportunity for *absentminded* injuries, so working with intention and full attention is an important aspect of our postural practice.

STRUGGLE CREATES STRESS

When we are in the stress response, the body releases a burst of adrenaline, making the heart rate and breath quicken, the pupils dilate, and the muscles contract to be ready for speed, giving us a burst of energy to escape danger. Inherently, that is beneficial for short periods of time but becomes a problem when it is a long-term chronic overdrive response. Our mindful yoga practice guides the nervous system out of the stress response into the rest/digest response, which slows the heart rate and the breath, and increases digestion and glandular activities supporting the immune system. It is important to catch yourself when you are pushing or struggling while practicing and pause to make another choice. This is a *no-pain* arena. If you feel pain or struggle in any way, stop what you are doing, breathe deeply, and reset.

Reset and return to clarity, feeling into what is needed, why you need it, and how to move forward as you guide your nervous system into a relaxation response.

Breathe deeply and slowly with intention. Focus on a positive outcome and intentions to harmonize the system. If the mind is wandering, distracted with the unconscious "What is going to happen to me?" or slipping into the "I need" mode, it keeps the nervous system in a chronic stress response. Our job is to consolidate and refine our thoughts to the essence of what is important to us.

Let your intentions guide the "how" of your practice. A practice driven by an intention to create *freedom* may feel different than a practice that is guided by the intention for *focus*. It's a consideration that does not need to be over-thought. Allow it to happen with a sense of curiosity and exploration.

Ahead is a guide to planting the seed of intention into the subconscious mind, cultivating a vow to ourselves, an inner declaration of sorts, to energize our journey. This works best when we cultivate it in a gentle repetition within a calm receptive mind. Tapping into our declaration and repeating it to inspire our poses creates fertile ground for the intention to become *actualization*.

I am healing.

Create a simple, straightforward declaration of your intention. Then fortify by visualizing the action and the positive outcome. Whatever you intend and envision, have it feel good when you think it, see it, and say it. With the vision, breathe into the emotion of how it feels, activating any sensory aspects of touch taste, smell, and sound. In this way, it becomes wired in the brain, and then our physical experience of pleasure follows suit. This is an example of neuro-connectivity, where we consciously create associations in the brain to hardwire the programming into our system. This can be a helpful or harmful association, this firing and wiring of the neuro-connections together, so we are consciously hardwiring pleasure into our vision of healing and growth. This hardwiring is connected to the Reticular Activating System (RAS) in our brain stem, which is our personal version of a homing device. This system will guide our mind to notice whatever we program it to. In simple terms, we can program it for pleasure, and we can program it to find pain. Ideally, we want to train the reticular activating system to help us find what we want by showing it what it looks, feels, and sounds like.

Setting intention at the beginning of the practice is one of the keys to its potency. This doesn't need to take significant time; as the habit becomes established, it may take as much time as a couple of breaths.

Conscious intention combined with the breath and skilled action creates transformation.

Pause now with me. Whether seated, standing, or reclined (as long as you aren't driving), close your eyes. Place a hand on the belly and a hand on the heart. Feel the weight of the hands on the torso. Breathe through the nose and feel the belly move out on the inhalation and in on the exhalation. The inhalation is the vehicle of cultivation, and exhalation is the vehicle of integration and surrender.

Use these inquiries to tap into your why and tune in to your intention. Consider creating a simple statement or declaration of one word for each inquiry, or the inquiry that speaks to you right now.

What am I healing or cultivating by doing this practice?
Use the inhalations to fulfill this intention.

Where am I making space or ease with this practice?
Use the exhalations to fulfill this intention.

Consider taking a few moments to breathe into the intention and to feel what it feels like to heal, to be free, to be happy in whatever it is.

Visualize what health looks like, what that sounds like, and that it is already so.

What is the one word or phrase that exemplifies my intention?

Keep it simple.
Write it down.
Say it out loud.

What you do every day will have the greatest impact on your health.

Now we have explored our why and have clarity on our intentions. Let's begin refining our physical template of steadiness and clarity. You began this exploration in the last chapter: how do you move or hold your body all day? How do you sit? Feet firmly planted, or do you tuck one foot under the other hip? How do you stand? Do you have one foot turned out with the hip shifted? Belly out and chin forward? How you align your body affects joint health and reveals a lot about your state of being and overall health.

Symmetry, steady and spacious in the body, creates balance in the mind. Direct your body and you will align your state of being.

Align your bones so the internal organs have space to do their job, your diaphragm muscle can support your breath, and the oxygen-rich blood can circulate with efficiency. For the next few days, observe your habitual patterns of sitting, standing, and sleeping. Log in your journal what you notice and consider what those patterns may create in the body and mind. If you are experiencing any pain or imbalances, can you see any direct or indirect connections with your habitual actions that could be contributing to your experience?

Right now, don't change anything; let's take a sample observance of your body position. Whether you are seated, standing or reclined, observe your body from the ground up.

Observe the Feet
Are they aligned in the same direction? Or different? Are they turned out, in, or straight ahead? If on the floor, where is the body weight centered? Center, inside, or outside of the foot? Forward toward the toes, or back toward the heels? How do they feel?

Observe the Legs and Hips
Are the legs aligned in the same direction? Or different? Are they turned out, in, or straight ahead? Where is the body weight in the pelvis? Centered, shifted forward toward pubic bone, back toward tailbone? Is the pelvis (or hips) rotated in any way? Is one side elevated higher than the other side? If so, which one? How do your low back and legs feel?

Observe the Upper Back, Shoulders, Neck, and Head
Are you hunched or rounded over? Are you upright with chest open? Are the shoulders rotated or straight ahead? Is one shoulder elevated higher than the other? If so, which one? What is the position of the neck and head? Are the chin, head, and neck jutted forward or pulled back? Are they centered with the neck in its natural curve? How do your upper back, shoulders, neck, and head feel?

The most efficient way to sit and stand is with the body in a neutral, symmetrically balanced spinal position. We often use the template of Mountain Pose, which is basically anatomical standing position. The spine, in its natural curve, supports all the body's functions, is energy-efficient, and supports clear thinking.

Like any structure, we look to the foundation to create stability and work our way up from that. If your feet are turned out or in and not neutral as in Mountain Pose, it creates imbalances that work their way up the entire body. Neck pain can have a root cause in the feet. Look from the ground up and begin to—lovingly, in a curious and nonjudgmental way—create symmetry and balance, like Mountain Pose, in your body every time you stand up. When seated, the sitting bones in the buttocks are the "feet" of your pelvis. Align them so the pelvis is upright and even on both sides (not rotated or elevated on either side). If your actual feet are on the floor, align both sets of feet, your feet and the pelvis's "feet." These simple shifts, practiced on a daily basis, will have big results and improve breathing, digestion, and cardiovascular and joint health. Consider adding this to your observation journal and log to see the tangible shifts you are creating.

Let's begin to explore some key asanas that create stability and clarity and support immune function. The immunity benefits of the postures in this chapter are listed below, and each posture will have additional benefits listed in the Particulars and Precautions section.

IMMUNITY AND WHOLE HEALTH BENEFITS OF THE FOLLOWING POSES

- Increases oxygenation/blood circulation.
- Aids in digestion, breathing, and cardiovascular, brain, and glandular function.
- Supports expansion of the diaphragm and the lungs.
- Decreases inflammation and aids in lymphatic drainage.
- Supports the rest/digest response of the parasympathetic nervous system.
- Supports mental/emotional outlook by releasing endorphins, serotonin, and dopamine.
- Supports homeostasis or whole-system balance.
- Supports self-regulation and connection into present-moment experience.
- Programs the Reticular Activating System (RAS) to aid in finding optimum circumstances for healing.
- Creates feelings of balance and clarity, and a calm, alert state.
- Activates vital energy (pranic) lines through the entire body.

POSES FOR CLARITY

TADASANA
(TA-DAH-SA-NA)
MOUNTAIN POSE

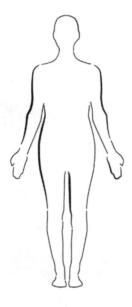

FOUNDATIONAL TEMPLATE FOR STABILITY AND BALANCE

Mountain Pose holds the key to all of the other poses and supports the body in an efficient, energized standard anatomical position. This standard position is the baseline template that supports us in standing tall, which we will compare all the other movements to. It's like the game Where's Waldo? Where is Mountain Pose? Where is it when you are sitting? Where is it when you are standing? Reclining? In another posture? Compare and contrast to see where there may be unconscious imbalances being created in the mind and body. Mountain Pose establishes a stable, symmetrical, joint and internal organ health baseline. Arms down or arms up, this pose creates balance, clarity, and intelligence in our actions, and is the blueprint for physical vitality.

STRETCHES (CREATING SPACE)

- Legs, torso, shoulders, and arms (Sun Stretch Series)
- Aids spinal and shoulder mobility (Sun Stretch Series)
- Creates space in torso/side waist, expanding lung capacity (Sun Stretch Series)

STRENGTHENS (CREATING STEADINESS)

- Feet, legs, core, spinal column, lungs, heart
- Supports a feeling of stability and a calm, alert, energized state

PARTICULARS AND PRECAUTIONS

- Can be used between other poses as a reset for the system.
- Can be done with back to a wall or seated erect on a chair for support.
- Use a block between the upper inner thighs to support low back and spine. (See exercise next page.)
- Full list of Immunity and Whole Health Benefits on page 44.

HOW TO DO IT

Breathe, connect with intention and visualize pose before doing.

- Align the feet hip-width apart and parallel.
- Spread the toes and press through from the mound of the big toe to the mound of the pinky toe while balancing the weight on inner to outer heel.
- Press down through the four markers of the feet while lifting up through inner and outer arches of the feet.
- Lift from the central arch of the feet to activate through the legs into the midline of the body.
- Lift the chest and widen evenly through all four sides of the torso and neck.
- Root down through the feet to rebound up through the rest of the body to stand tall.

- Once tall, relax and hang from the crown of the head, as if there were a cosmic puppeteer holding the body up by an etheric cord, creating a calm alert state.
- Breathe evenly, cultivating balance and clarity of purpose, before moving to another posture.

A point of interest: Energizing through the arches of the feet and the centers of the palms stimulates key pranic or energetic points in the body, called *marma* points, which stimulate all the other energy channels. You are truly waking up your whole body!

STANDING PELVIC FLOOR EXERCISE (ENHANCES STABILITY AND SPINAL INTEGRITY)

The perineum or pelvic floor is essential to core stability and to spinal, reproductive, and digestive elimination health.

Utilizing a yoga block, place it between the thighs up high, away from the knees (if the block were a piece of Pez candy, it would shoot forward). While standing, hold the block in place and press down through the four pillars of the feet: big toe mound, pinky toe mound, inner and outer heel. As you anchor the four pillars, lift up through the inner/outer arches of the feet, drawing up through the arches and activating the inner thighs as you squeeze the block. Inhale while you soften the legs and pelvic floor (the urine-stopping muscle between genital and anus). Exhale, squeeze, and contract in and up through feet, legs, and pelvic floor. Pull up into the navel and continue to elongate through the spine to the crown of the head. Repeat eight times. Do three sets.

SUN STRETCH SERIES

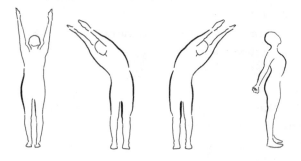

INSPIRED LIFT, SUN STRETCHES, AND C-CLASP

PARTICULARS AND PRECAUTIONS

- Appropriate for any time of day, but avoid before bedtime.
- Can be used between other poses to invigorate and reset the system.
- Add block between the thighs, as on page 47, to support core and spinal column.
- Widen the arms, creating space in shoulders and neck, if there is strain.
- Full list of Immunity and Whole Health Benefits on page 44.

HOW TO DO IT

- Start standing in Mountain Pose.
- Inhale, with a clear intention of creating vitality and inspiration, and reach arms out around and above the head.
- From the shoulder socket, rotate the arms and palms to face each other and make space around the neck.
- Relax the neck and shrugging muscles.
- Energize up by rooting into the feet and rebounding through whole body up to the sky.
- Visualize a V or downward-pointing triangle pouring warm sunlight down into your belly button and open wide on top from the chest through the arms.

- Pause, standing tall, radiating up to the sky.
- Breathe deeply to energize, closing or softening the eyes to imagine connecting into the sun's radiance.
- When ready, proceed to lateral side stretches.

LATERAL SIDE STRETCHES

- Stretch the arms up and over to one side, gently tucking the chin to create mild pressure on the thyroid and thymus glands in and near the throat.
- Inhale slowly and come back up to central, arms still reaching up, and slowly repeat lateral side stretch to the other side.
- Return to center, creating that brilliant V shape to the sky, firm the belly, and stay lifted until there is a physical, mental, and emotional shift. Lower the arms, preparing to clasp hands behind the back for a C-Clasp stretch.

TRANSITION INTO C-CLASP (HANDS-BEHIND-THE-BACK STRETCH)

- With arms down, stabilize the stance from the feet up through the rest of the body.
- Reach the arms behind the back, turning the arms and palms to face each other to link the thumbs, or utilize a towel or strap.
- Straighten through the elbows, creating long arms and wrists, while you lift the chest up and stretch.
- If the elbows bend and will not straighten, add a strap, tie, or towel— something to add length and width to the hands before deepening.
- Breathe balanced breaths for three to five rounds before releasing hands and arms along the sides of the torso.
- Consider placing the palms together at the chest center, pressing the heels of the hands together, and bringing the forearms parallel to the floor to complete the energizing and clarity process before moving on, or repeating this series until you feel clear and inspired.

Sun stretches can also be practiced seated on a chair or reclined, first supine and then prone, to accommodate all movements.

UTKATASANA
(OOK-AH-TAS-SA-NA)
THUNDERBOLT OR CHAIR POSE

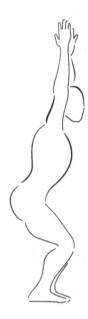

STABILITY, ENDURANCE, CLARITY, STRENGTHENS LEGS/BUTTOCKS

When we take a stably held "seat," we create whole-being strength. To the jovial groans of my students, this is one of the most-utilized clarity postures in my classes because it quickly moves attention into the body and moves energy into focusing on what is needed. It has low risks and high benefits, and can be modified for most bodies to create balance, strength, focus, and thunderbolt clarity.

STRETCHES (CREATING SPACE)

- Hips, spine; opens chest and shoulders
- Relieves lower back compression and backaches

STRENGTHENS (CREATING STEADINESS)

- Feet, legs, buttocks, core, spinal column, lungs, heart, shoulders (arms up)
- Builds strength, stamina, and balance

PARTICULARS AND PRECAUTIONS

- Creates heat in the body.
- Can be practiced anytime, but avoid before bedtime.
- Can be used between other poses to increase or maintain heat and focus.
- Practice with back to a wall for balance support.
- Add block between the thighs, as on page 47, to support core and spinal column.
- Deepen angle of knee bend to increase effort and challenge. Stop at the maximum of ninety degrees, knee directly over the ankle. Never take knee past a right angle.
- Avoid if there are acute knee problems or frailty; if high blood pressure, consider keeping hands on the hips.
- Full list of Immunity and Whole Health Benefits page 44.

HOW TO DO IT

Breathe, connect with intention, and visualize pose before doing.

- Align the feet hip-width apart and parallel to each other.
- Bend the knees, drawing the weight of the body back toward the heels into a sustainable elevated seat.
- Lift up from the belly and lengthen the chest and head while reaching arms upwards.
- Continue to cultivate a balance of effort: stable and relaxed.
- Hold for five breaths, stand up, and repeat if desired (and feels helpful).

Pay attention to knee position! Stack the knees directly over the ankles and track the knees in line with the second toe of the foot. Do not allow the knees to go past the ankles or lean side to side, as it can cause strain and injury.

TRANSITION INTO CHAIR POSE CAT/COW (ARCH/ROUND THE SPINE)

Increase spinal mobility and circulation with arching and rounding the spine in Chair Pose.

- Starting in Chair Pose, hinge the torso forward into a diagonal from legs.
- Inhale, then pull the chest forward, widening the chest and arching the spine.
- Exhale, tuck the chin, firm the belly, and round the spine.
- Repeat on the breath, arching then rounding the spine, from three to six times.
- When complete, slowly return to standing or progress to the twist.

TRANSITION INTO CHAIR POSE TWIST

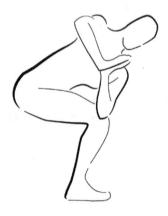

- Increase spinal mobility, rejuvenate spinal discs, and enhance digestion with spinal rotation in this twisted variation of Chair Pose.
- Start in Chair Pose with the weight toward the heels.
- Lengthen through the entire torso and reach up through the arms.
- Engage core muscles, draw the navel toward the spine, and turn the chest to the left; bring the arms down and utilize the right hand or elbow on the outside of the left thigh for leverage.
- Stabilize the legs/hips and focus the twist into the upper back.
- Inhale, lengthen through the spine; exhale, deepen the twist.
- Allow head to go along for the ride and follow the rotation led by the chest.
- The chest center leads, and the head follows.
- Hold each side from three to six breath cycles or as long as you feel stable and spacious.
- Stop in the center and stabilize between sides.
- When both sides are complete, slowly return to standing or shift into Standing Forward Fold to reset and then proceed deeper into the practice.

In spinal twists, in yoga and in life, ideally, the heart leads and the head is to follow.

UTTANASANA
(OOT-A-NAH-SA-NA)
STANDING FORWARD FOLD

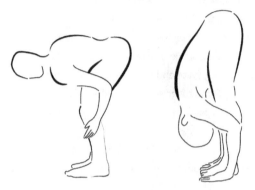

CALMING, SPINAL RELEASE, MASSAGES ABDOMEN, STRETCHES LEGS

This standing forward fold can create a satisfying stretch in the back of the legs as well as a soothing, cooling effect on the nervous system. The nature of a forward fold is to gently massage the internal organs and draw awareness inside to create calm. For some, however, a deep forward fold can feel confining and confrontational. Explore this posture with a sense of slow curiosity. Do not push the fold by rounding the spine, or tucking the chin to press the face into the legs—instead, lengthen through the front of the torso, keeping the spine long and chest open as you hinge from the hips. Start with the knees bent to facilitate a long, even spine and a feeling of openness as you, over time, gently work deeper into the fold.

STRETCHES (CREATING SPACE)

- Stretches the back of legs, hips, buttocks, spine
- Massages internal organs and abdomen

STRENGTHENS (CREATING STEADINESS)

- Strengthens feet, legs, and core
- Supports a feeling of stability and calmness

Start the pose with bent knees. Place the hands on the outside of the shins, elbows drawn back, pressing the belly into thighs to massage internal organs and breathe deeply as preparation for going into the full pose.

PARTICULARS AND PRECAUTIONS

- Cools and calms the body.
- Increases lung expansion and air circulation in the back of the lungs.
- Appropriate any time of day or evening.
- Can be practiced between other poses to calm and reset the system.
- Bend the knees if strain in the low back.
- Place hands on block or outside of the shins for stability and to create space in the low back.
- Avoid if you have spinal disc issues or sciatic pain.
- Full list of Immunity and Whole Health Benefits page 44.

HOW TO DO IT

Breathe, connect with intention, and visualize pose before doing.

- Start in Chair or Mountain Pose, bend the knees, and hinge from the hips to fold, pressing the lower belly to the top of the thighs.
- Shift the body weight slightly forward into the balls of the feet, allowing neck to relax.
- Press belly onto the thighs, keeping knees bent and lengthening through the spine.
- Stretch the chest away from the hips, with hands on shins, blocks, or floor.
- Avoid rounding the upper back.
- Lengthen through the front body, navel to head.
- Stack hips over the heels; avoid dropping the hips back.
- Press belly onto the thighs while slowly straightening the legs.
- Go very slow and do not force the legs to straighten.
- Slow and steady, daily gentle stretching will reap inspiring results.

VIRABHADRASANA 2
(VEER-A-BAH-DRAHS-AH-NA)
WARRIOR 2 POSE

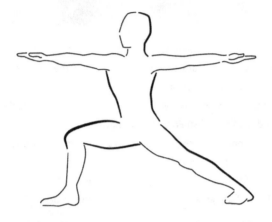

STABILIZES, CREATES ENDURANCE, STRENGTHENS LEGS

Accessible to most, this standing pose is a cornerstone of this clarity asana practice. It builds strength, stability, and openness, all at the same time. It can be readily modified to increase focus and challenge by simply widening the stance and increasing the depth of the front knee. The root name, Vira, is often referred to as "warrior" and yet it also can be translated into courage. Consider highlighting the peaceful courage of this posture which, with its deep anchor into the legs and earth, helps us rise up in clarity and create courage for what is important to us. Practicing this pose can help you bring energy to your wellness practices as well as your whole life.

STRETCHES (CREATING SPACE)

- Hips, groin, spine, opens chest and shoulders
- Relieves lower back compression and backaches

STRENGTHENS (CREATING STEADINESS)

- Feet, legs, buttocks, core, spinal column, lungs, heart, shoulders
- Builds strength, stamina, and balance

PARTICULARS AND PRECAUTIONS

- Creates heat in the body.
- Can be practiced anytime, but avoid before bedtime.
- Keep front knee stacked and tracked over the ankle to avoid injury.
- Practice with back to a wall or seated erect on a chair for balance support.
- Avoid if acute knee problems or extreme frailty.
- Full list of Immunity and Whole Health Benefits, page 44.

HOW TO DO IT

Breathe, connect with intention, and visualize pose before doing.

- Open the arms out to the side, step the feet under the wrists or fingertips, whichever is most stable.
- From the hip socket, rotate the leg bone so the foot and knee are aligned forward.
- Create heel-to-back-arch alignment with the feet.
- Stack knee over the ankle, aligned with the second toe of foot.
- Lengthen up through side waist so the torso is even on all sides.
- Inhale, then reach the arms out to the side, parallel to the earth and palms turned up.
- Breathe evenly through the nose, while holding gaze toward the front hand.
- Hold as long as you feel steady, balanced, energized, and relaxed simultaneously.
- Step back to center, creating Mountain Pose, then do the other side.
- Always do both sides, balancing equal time with equal intensity.

BALASANA
(BA-LAH-SA-NA)
CHILD'S POSE

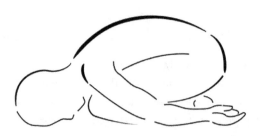

RESETS, CALMS, RELEASES HIPS/LOW BACK

A pose that is dedicated to non-doing. A return to surrender and inner sanctuary as an innocent babe sleeping, curled into a ball. I can clearly remember each of my littles sound asleep with their baby bums slightly up in the air. Allow this pose to have its feel-good effects effortlessly. When the thighs are pressed together, it creates an abdominal massage, supporting elimination and toning the diaphragm. When the legs are slightly apart, it releases the abdominals and diaphragm. If the intense flexion puts too much pressure on the knees, place a rolled bath towel between the buttocks and the calves to help relieve it. This pose is like salt and pepper, it can be added to any yoga meal when needed to bring the system back to balance.

STRETCHES (CREATING SPACE)

- Stretches the front of the legs, hips, buttocks, lower back, shoulders, neck
- Massages internal organs and abdomen

STRENGTHENS (CREATING STEADINESS)

- Relaxation and reset of whole body
- Supports a feeling of stability and calmness

- Cools and calms the entire system.
- Appropriate any time of day or evening.
- Can be used between other poses as a reset for the system.
- Excellent pose to tone diaphragm and lungs practicing Full Complete Pranayama, page 77.
- Add padding under the knees or to the back of the knees if strain.
- Separate thighs if pregnant or strain on diaphragm or throat.
- Avoid if acute knee problems or extreme frailty.
- Full list of Immunity and Whole Health Benefits, page 44.

HOW TO DO IT

Breathe, connect with intention, and visualize pose before doing.

- Starting on all fours, exhale to draw the hips back toward the heels, inhaling to create space through the spine and outer hips.
- Separate knees slightly and draw the big toes together to touch.
- Inhale to lengthen the sides of the torso.
- Exhale to relax the head, shoulders, and hips toward the floor.
- Breath in and out through the nose, expanding the low belly and relaxing the entire system.

Rest the forehead on the forearms or a yoga block if the head does not comfortably rest on the floor.

ADHO MUKHA SHVANASANA
(AH-DOH-MOO-KHA-SHVAH-NAH-SA-NA)
DOWNWARD-FACING DOG

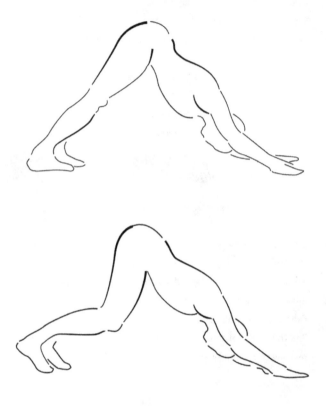

SURRENDER, STABILITY, SPINAL LENGTH, STRETCHES BACK OF LEGS

Down Doggy is the quintessential yoga posture for the modern age. This poster image of an active yoga practice can be a resting pose, and, in the beginning, it is not easy. You may have heard a yoga teacher kindly say, "Rest in Down Dog," and felt like you were working the hardest! Start with short holds and with the knees fully bent. Even if you are seasoned at this posture, start this way to tilt the pelvis and release the spine, which is our first priority here, reversing the effects of gravity on the spinal discs and internal organs and creating traction for the neck.

STRETCHES (CREATING SPACE)

- Stretches the back of legs, calves, hips, buttocks, spine, shoulders, arms and hands
- Stretches intercostals and reduces spinal compression effects of gravity
- Massages internal organs and abdomen

STRENGTHENS (CREATING STEADINESS)

- Strengthens hands, arms, shoulders, core, spine, legs and feet
- Supports a feeling of stability, surrender, and calmness

PARTICULARS AND PRECAUTIONS

- Can be cooling or heating, depending on practitioner.
- Appropriate any time of day or evening.
- Can be practiced between other poses to calm and reset the system.
- Bend the knees if any strain in the low back.
- Turn hands slightly out and wider than shoulder-width if shoulders and neck are tight.
- Utilize forearms instead of hands if there is a wrist issue.
- Add block between the thighs, as on page 47, to support core and spinal column.
- Avoid if hiatal hernia, high or low blood pressure, history of stroke, or glaucoma or detached retina.
- Full list of Immunity and Whole Health Benefits, page 44.

> Start the pose with the knees bent and heels lifted to facilitate the hips moving fully up and back to create traction for the entire spinal column.

Breathe, connect with intention, and visualize pose before doing.

- Start in Child's Pose and stretch arms forward, placing hands on the floor shoulder-width apart.
- Press and spread evenly through palms and fingers, opening them like a sunburst.
- Root between the thumb and index finger on both hands and activate the forearms up from the floor.
- Draw the forearms toward each other until there is stability in the shoulders and neck.
- Shift the hips up and back with the knees bent, elongating through the spine.
- Allow the head to hang and create traction through the hips, spine, neck, and head.
- Firm the belly and stabilize the body so that the breath can be conscious and relaxed.
- Release tension by gently turning the head side to side, chew through the jaw, and massage through the feet and calves while keeping the knees bent.
- Stretch and lengthen the entire spine.
- Slowly straighten the legs and lengthen heels toward the floor (no need for them to touch!).
- If the spine rounds, rebend the knees, as the spinal length is the priority.
- Breathe smoothly and hold as long as sustainable without struggle.
- Return to Child's Pose.

PHALAKASANA
(FA-LAH-KAHS-A-NA)
PLANK POSE

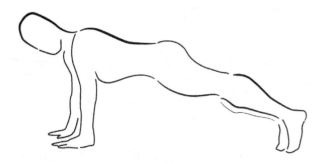

FOCUS, CONFIDENCE. STRENGTHENS ENTIRE BODY

As if you plugged your heels into a metaphorical electrical socket, this pose energizes, clarifies, and strengthens mind, body, and spirit. Create an arrow of intention with the heart, eyes, and whole body while breathing and holding the body up over the floor. Floating between earth and sky, this posture is a fantastic mix of physical and heart consciousness work. It is potent, so no need to overdo it—build strength in a spacious way, without struggle. Catch yourself when you are pushing or punishing yourself in some way, take the struggle out of the pose, and practice it with a sense of positive possibility and pleasure.

STRETCHES (CREATING SPACE)

- Stretches the back of legs, calves, hips, buttocks, spine, shoulders, arms and hands

STRENGTHENS (CREATING STEADINESS)

- Strengthens hands, arms, shoulders, back, core, spine, legs and feet
- Supports a feeling of focus, stability, clarity and confidence

PARTICULARS AND PRECAUTIONS

- Creates heat in the body.
- Appropriate any time; avoid evening and before bedtime.
- Can be practiced between other poses to create heat and focus.
- Utilize forearms instead of hands if there is a wrist issue.
- Add block between the thighs, as in page 44, to support core and spinal column.
- Press the heels into a wall to activate the legs and take weight off the upper body.
- Avoid this posture if you have wrist or shoulder issues or if frail.
- Full list of Immunity and Whole Health Benefits, page 47.

Consider starting the pose in half-plank, with the knees resting on the floor, and building the alignment and strength to hold the full posture.

HOW TO DO IT

Breathe, connect with intention, and visualize pose before doing.

- Start in Downward-Facing Dog or extended Child's Pose, with the hands shoulder-width apart.
- Stack shoulders directly over the wrists.
- Press the thighs up to align the hips with the shoulders, creating a long line from the heels to the crown of the head.
- Gaze just slightly forward to support length on all four sides of the neck.
- Firm the belly and press back through the heels as you pull the chest slightly forward to lengthen body in opposite directions.
- Relax the breath while holding the posture, and pay attention to any gripping or overworking in the body, especially the face, jaw, and buttocks. Soften those.
- Hold for a minimum of three breaths, to a maximum of fifteen— don't go beyond what feels steady and relaxed. Transition back to Downward-Facing Dog or Child's Pose.

CHAPTER 3

PRANAYAMA FOR CLARITY

Breath is life. It is the last thing to come as we are birthed into this world and the first thing to go when we leave. We can't stay in our bodies without it. The movement of the diaphragm muscle contracting down into the abdominal cavity and then releasing back up creates a vacuum that moves the air in and out of the lungs. It also massages the internal organs, stirring all that fluid in the lower cavity. This mushroom-like dome is a key circulator in our body, supporting the lungs, heart, and digestion.

Close the mouth and take a slow deep breath through the nose. Inhale through the nose, expanding down deep into the abdomen and belly, exhale back through the nose, feel the belly release. Continue to repeat as we explore here.

The nose and sinuses clear the air. Use your nose to take in the breath, as it is a key valve that filters the air of debris (including bacteria and viruses) and warms and humidifies the air for our lungs. The movement through the sinuses can also be calming to our nervous system and support overall health. Use the mouth to breathe only for a specific breath exercise or when talking, train yourself to inhale nearly all of the time through your nose.

As we inhale, the diaphragm muscle essentially splits the abdomen into two parts, lungs above for air and the bottom part for the fluid-filled balloons of the intestinal tract. Along the diaphragm's back attachments near the back ribs, it connects with the sprawling vagus nerve, whose main function (if you recall from Chapter 1) is to calm us down and stimulate our immune system. When fully expanded, the diaphragm's posterior attachments stimulate the vagus nerve and signals the brain stem that we are breathing deeply, which means we are safe. What do we do when we are stressed or in danger? We hold our breath and take shallow, quick breaths. It works reciprocally here; if we perceive danger, which causes us stress, we breathe shallowly. If we breathe in small quick breaths, our nervous system perceives danger, and all our energy goes toward running from the tiger versus living to a ripe old age. The opposite is also true. If we breathe deeply, with slow, full breaths, our nervous system perceives safety. The mind is peaceful and the body breathes expansive breaths.

Shallow Quick Breaths = Danger	Perceived Danger = Depressed Immune Function
Deep Slow Breathes = Safety	Perceived Safety = Boosted Immune Function

REST/DIGEST BENEFITS

- Helps the mind/body feel safe and increases energy for longevity functions.
- Longevity functions are immunity, hormone function, and digestion/elimination.
- Increases oxygenation of the blood and circulation.
- Decreases stress hormones such as cortisol.
- Decreases systemic inflammation.
- Softens muscular tension and reduces pain sensation.
- Enhances mental/cognitive function, clarity, and concentration.
- Increases resilience and emotional balance.
- Enhances ability to stay in present-moment experience, therefore building the ability to be more mindful.

Deep breaths open the lungs and clear stale air. When bacteria and viruses get cozy in the far-reaching areas of our lungs, where there is little movement to disturb them or move them out, it spells trouble. Chronic shallow breathing, poor spinal alignment, and stressed-out, sluggish immune function really spells trouble.

Our job is to get that diaphragm muscle toned and habitually expanding to its full capacity to move fresh air into those far-reaching parts of the lungs, clear out the muck, and with the movement, circulate fresh blood deep into all the crevices of the body for renewal. Because many of us breathe shallow breaths, we are in a chronic stress response. We need to get our lungs activated to boost our immune system and rejuvenate our pulmonary system. Cultivating healthy lungs, a strong diaphragm and vagal tonality are the big items on this chapter's to-do list.

The exercises that follow teach you how to consciously stimulate the vagus nerve to push that magic relaxation button for yourself (and create a habit of doing that all day long) and move oxygen and fresh air deep into the back of the lungs. Later, in the upcoming chapters, we will go deeper into spring-cleaning the depths of the lungs. Each of these tools build on each other to help boost immunity.

Breathing exercises move vital life force through our physical bodies. In the yoga tradition, that vital life force that animates all life is called *prana*; in Chinese healing and martial arts, *qi* or *chi*. The essential animating force of pure energy that is life, we in yoga call prana. Our mind, our movement of the body, and our breathing directly affects the quality of our prana and therefore how we feel. Whether we feel *tamasic* (sluggish and dull), *rajasic* (hyper and agitated), or *sattvic* (balanced and in harmony), it is all about our energies of prana. Breathing practices directly affect our pranic quality and therefore are called *pranayama* (PRAH-na-YAH-ma).

Prana = Life Force | Yama = To Direct
The conscious act of directing the breath and life force to bring balance and harmony to the system.

The self-study and poses help prepare us for the more subtle and advanced practices of *pranayama* (energy awareness and conscious breathing). Many of the breathing exercises are done with a still body, either seated or reclined. It takes a stable, relatively pain-free body and calm mind to be still, so consistently do your practice to expand your capacities and experience of whole health.

PREPARING FOR BREATHING EXERCISES AND MEDITATION

We prepare to sit by moving, stretching and strengthening the body, and getting clear on our intentions. Once the body and the mind feel steady and spacious enough to be still, then we are ready for the next potent layer of the yogic practices, the *pranayamas* and meditations. The direct translation of *asana* is actually not posture, like Down Dog, but steady and spacious *seat*, like a meditation seat. Over time, that meaning has shifted to include many various physical postures, and yet the original meaning is our guide here. The seat is what we will utilize to breathe, heal the body, focus the mind, and merge with our essential self.

QUESTION COMFORTABLE

Is this position going to be sustainable in stillness for the next five, ten, twenty minutes? When I teach new yoga teachers, we talk about the word "comfortable" and why we avoid using this word when guiding yoga students. Comfort is very subjective. I tease them and slump like a sack of potatoes in my seat, miming holding a TV remote, looking drowsy. Upper back humped, head jutted forward, body in a heap. I then say," This is very comfortable, is this good for practice?" Knowing that in a very short amount of time that posture will lead me to dullness, discomfort and pain, they exclaim "No!" What is valuable here is a steady upright seat, which means one that supports the functions of the body for the long term, right and left sides of the body in symmetry and the natural curvature of the spine lifted. This steadiness may not feel the most comfortable in the beginning simply because the body may not be used to aligning and holding in this way. That is okay. That is part of our work to build a healthier body that is steady and spacious.

CREATE STEADY/SPACIOUS

Cultivate a sense of effortlessness in holding the pranayama posture. If you are struggling in any way, then the mind will be hooked onto that effort and not relax. In this way, guide yourself to choose a posture, either seated or reclined, that is sustainable long-term. Each day is different, so allow for the flexibility to shift the postures you practice in each day, as determined by your physical and mental state of being. Trust your body to tell you what will be the most sustainable for today.

SUPPORTED SUKHASANA
(SOO-KAH-SA-NA)
CROSS-LEGGED SEAT ON A LIFT

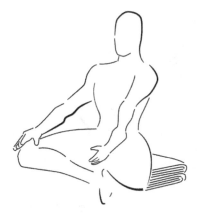

HIPS ON A SUPPORT LIFTED HIGHER THAN THE KNEES

Come to a cross-legged position, sitting on the floor with the hips higher than the knees. For most bodies, it is ideal to sit on a support (yoga block, firm pillow, folded blankets) to lift the hips higher than the knees, similar to a tetrahedron shape. This helps release the low back, take strain off the knees, and reduce nerve compression that results in pins and needles.

Once the hips are lifted, align the body in symmetry on both sides with length and support for the natural curvature of the spine. It can be helpful to use the support of a wall behind the back for longer holds.

Bring awareness to the pelvis and create a slight tilt of body weight forward toward the pubic bone (versus the weight back onto the tailbone). Gently lift abdominal muscles in and up to draw support into the upper back, drawing it in toward the chest. Lift and broaden the chest, stabilizing the neck curve to support the head being upright with ears in line with the shoulders (versus chin jutted forward).

SUPPORTED VAJRASANA
(VAJ-RAH-SA-NA)
KNEELING SEAT ON A LIFT

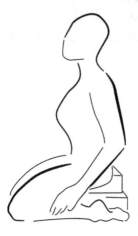

Come to kneeling on the floor (or with padding such as a blanket under the knees) with the hips lifted higher than the knees. For most bodies, it is ideal to sit on a support (yoga block, firm pillow, folded blankets) to lift the hips higher than the knees. This helps release the low back, take strain off the knees and reduce nerve compression that results in pins and needles. Once hips are lifted, align the body in symmetry on both sides with length and support for the natural curvature of the spine. Bring awareness to the pelvis and create a slight tilt of body weight forward toward the pubis versus back on the tailbone. Gently lift abdominal muscles in and up to draw support into the upper back drawing it in toward the chest. Lift and broaden the chest stabilizing the neck curve to support the head being upright with ears in line with the shoulder's (versus chin jutted forward).

PROPER UPRIGHT SEAT ON A CHAIR

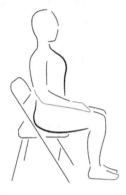

Come to sit on a firm upright chair with the feet anchored to the ground, feet hip-width and parallel to each other, with the knees stacked right over the heels. Shift forward if necessary to ensure the sitting bones are evenly anchored to the seat and there is a slight shift forward to the pelvis, where a little more weight is toward the pubis versus back on the tailbone. This helps release the low back, take strain off the knees, and reduce nerve compression that results in pins and needles. Gently lift abdominal muscles in and up to draw support into the upper back, drawing it in toward the chest. Lift and broaden the chest, stabilizing the neck curve to support the head being upright with ears in line with the shoulders (versus chin jutted forward).

SUPINE AND PRONE

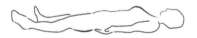 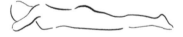

Come to lie either supine on the back or prone on the belly. Use any blankets or props to support release of the body and support of the natural curvature of the spine. If prone, turn the head to rest on one ear, even out the next time by switching to the other ear to create balance on both sides. These are very good postures if the system is weakened or fatigued in any way. The pro here is ease and the con is the tendency for the mind and body to fall asleep. Although that may feel counterproductive to the desire to practice conscious breathing and meditation, I want to support you giving yourself that sleep with appreciation and generosity, as many of us are sleep-deprived (which we will discuss more in Chapter 5). Sleeping is one of the essentials in supporting the longevity functions, the immune system, as well as a happy life, and as one of my favorite yoga teachers, Indu Arora, says, "Make sleep a priority!" So, if you nod off in practice, consider it a blessing.

SUPINE WITH BENT KNEES

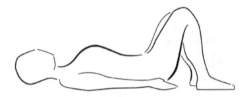

Create more ease by reclining supine on the back, knees bent with feet on the floor. This releases effort on the spinal column and is accessible for most bodies and times of life.

PRONE ON THE BELLY

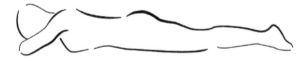

Utilize the weight of the body and the resistance of the floor to expand back body awareness. On the belly creates a grounded feeling and helps create greater openness in the back of the lungs and around the the vagus nerve.

BEST PRACTICES FOR BREATHING EXERCISES

If possible, empty the bladder and bowels before practicing and, ideally, practice pranayama on an empty stomach. Avoid drinking water during practice, yet proper hydration before and after is recommended. The most potent times to practice are before sunrise or after sunset, in the quieter, cooler times of day. Once the body is stable, practice pranayama with the eyes closed to draw the awareness inward to the subtleties.

Avoid pushing or straining with any part of the breath. Less is truly more in this situation, as it is better to do a few to start and do them with ease than to do many, programming struggle into the system. It is normal to fall asleep in the beginning. Practice will grow the ability to hold attention; if falling asleep feels like an issue, choose an upright seat for your practices.

BREATH RATIOS

A note on breath length, retentions, and ratios. The use of ratios to guide pranayama is a yogic standard. 1:1 is a ratio of inhalation to exhalation. This is shorthand for guiding the breath and is used in many of the breathing exercises throughout this book. 1:1 is one inhalation to one exhalation. 4:4 is a 4-count inhalation to a 4-count exhalation. 4:1 is a 4-count inhalation to a much shorter 1-count exhalation. Each ratio offers a different benefit and effect which, when utilized, will be described in the exercises. When the breath is intentionally paused or held, it is called a retention. Generally, retentions are considered a more advanced practice, and different types and lengths of retentions have different effects on attention and the movement of energy.

When retentions are involved in ratios it looks like this 1:1:1:1

1 inhalation

to

1 retention hold

to

1 exhalation

to

1 retention hold

Later, in Chapter 11, you will be directed to a 5:5:5:5 breath ratio, which is a 5-count inhalation, 5-count retention (held breath in), 5-count exhalation, and 5-count retention (held breath out).

The above are simply some best practices, so do not let them deter you. The foundational breathing that we share in this chapter can be practiced most any time of day and in any position, although the best experience will be obtained where the body is in symmetry, even on both sides, the natural curvature of the spine is supported with little to no effort in holding the body in position, and the mind is easily able to focus on the breath, which will shift your vital energy and boost your life.

The experience is in the doing and feeling, so let's get breathing!

All of the breathing exercises here begin with a full and natural exhalation and then the next direct inhalation. We are using a conscious reset as the initiation into the movement of the pranayama or direction of pranic life force through breathing.

With each exercise, tune in to higher intention and to enhance mindful initiation of the breath. Remember what you are cultivating, and that it brings nourishment to your body and life. Intention moves life force and is the power behind pranayama.

IMMUNITY AND WHOLE HEALTH BENEFITS OF FOLLOWING EXERCISES

- Increases oxygen intake and decreases carbon dioxide/debris/stale air.
- Increases blood oxygen and lymphatic and digestive circulation.
- Increase lung/diaphragm strength and elasticity.
- Decreases stress overdrive functions, heart rate, blood pressure, and inflammation.
- Stimulates the vagus nerve, activating the rest/digest response (description on page 66).
- Mindful repetitions support the slowing of brain waves and calming the mind.
- Cultivates present-moment awareness, supporting focus, concentration, mental/emotional balance.
- Supports self-regulation, resilience, endurance, and whole-system balance.
- Reduces anxiety, depression, fatigue, brain fog, and feelings of overwhelm.
- With intention, focuses the reticular activation system (RAS) on positive healing outcome.
- Activates vital energy currents in the body, increasing health, vitality, and radiance.

PRACTICES FOR CLARITY

SAMA VRITTI
(SAH-MA VREE-TEE)
BALANCED 1:1 RATIO BREATHING

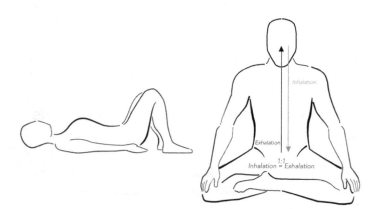

FOUNDATIONAL, GROUNDING, BALANCE, CALMING

Yogis understand that the quality of the breath is directly related to the quality of the mind, and I have definitely had direct experience with this over the years. This is a key to health and happiness. When the length of the inhalation is balanced with the length of the exhalation, the mind begins to quiet and the nervous system calms. Sama Vritti or Balanced Ratio Breathing directly and positively affects immune function and is a foundational practice for all levels of practitioner, used any time of day.

PARTICULARS AND PRECAUTIONS

- Cultivates focus, balance, and relaxation.
- Appropriate any time of day/evening,
- Utilized alone, in asana, and in life activities as a system balancer.
- Full list of Immunity and Whole Health Benefits page 44.

Stabilize body, elongate spine, cultivating balance; sitting or reclined position can be used.

- Direct the breath out the nostrils; upon inhalation, feel the coolness of the air in the nasal openings.
- Exhale the breath completely out.
- Inhale through the nose while calmly noting the length of the breath, creating a sustainable fullness.
- Guide the exhalation out the nostrils for the same length and quality.
- Cultivate *sama*, or balanced inhale and exhalations, for the entirety of the repetitions.
- Begin with a 1:1 ratio and slowly expand length to 3:3, 4:4, and 5:5.

FULL COMPLETE BREATHS
BELLY OR DIAPHRAGMATIC BREATHING

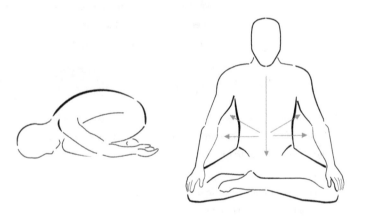

FOUNDATIONAL, GROUNDING, BALANCE, OPENS BACK OF
DIAPHRAGM/LUNGS

Using a Full Complete breath or Diaphragmatic Belly Breath to expand lung elasticity in the often-neglected distal posterior areas of the lungs. Average modern living cultivates compressed, slumped body position (remember the image of sitting like a sack of potatoes in a heap holding the remote?), producing chronic shallow breathing which not only creates a chronic stress response, but also minimally activates the anterior superior areas of the lungs. Think of chest breathing or shallow panting. Here we will activate all areas of the lungs, including both distal and posterior, to optimize immune support and feel as if we have opened up shuttered windows on a clear spring day.

PARTICULARS AND PRECAUTIONS

- Cultivates focus, balance, and relaxation.
- Expands often-neglected side/back areas of the lungs.
- Appropriate any time of day/evening.
- Utilized alone, in asana, and in life activities as a system balancer.
- Good in postures where spine is supported and core engagement is not needed; avoid in vigorous asanas.
- Full Complete breath demands a relaxation of the stabilizing pelvic floor and lower abdominal muscles, so it is not appropriate for active asana or any body movement where spinal stabilization is needed.
- Full list of Immunity and Whole Health Benefits page 44.

HOW TO DO IT

Stabilize body, elongate spine, cultivating balance; sitting or reclined position can be used, although a Forward Fold or Child's Pose with belly compression may help make the breath more accessible.

- Direct the breath out the nostrils, upon inhalation, feel the coolness of the air in the nasal openings.
- Inhale through the nose while calmly noting the length of the breath, creating a sustainable fullness.
- Guide the exhalation out the nostrils for the same length and quality.
- Focus on expanding the lower belly region under the navel with the inhalation. Imagine that you are blowing up a bicycle tire expand the

breath in front under the navel, along the lower side waist, and then all the way back around to the back bottom ribs.

- Stretching open the diaphragm muscle and its attachments where it is connected to the front, sides, and the back of the rib cage, again as if you are blowing up a bicycle tire.
- Refine by pressing the hands on the side ribs and, as you breathe, pushing them out, away from the body. Do this as many times as needed to feel connected to this expansion.
- Lower the hands to press just under the back bottom ribs, above the low back, near the kidney area. Create steady firm pressure (not so much there is any discomfort) there as you inhale to fully expand the front, sides, and back of the diaphragm attachments.
- Once this full front, side, back breathing is cultivated, then focus to expand the length of the breaths, as long as there is no push or strain.
- Cultivate *sama* or balanced inhale and exhalations for the entirety of the repetitions.
- Begin with 4:4 ratio and slowly expand length to 5:5, 6:6, and possibly beyond, as long as no strain.

EXPANSIVE THREE-PART DIAPHRAGMATIC BREATHING

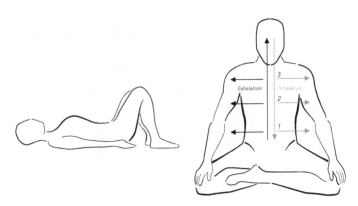

GENTLY INVIGORATING, BALANCING, DEEPLY OPENS BACK OF DIAPHRAGM/LUNGS

Expansive Three-part Diaphragmatic Breathing builds on a Full Complete breath, continuing the opening of the abdominal cavity to include the thoracic (mid-torso) as well as clavicular (upper torso into throat) areas of the body. We are building on the ability and awareness to expand the lower belly and the diaphragm attachments upon the inhalation, and then drawing that expansion slowly, breath by breath, into the mid-chest thoracic area and finally into the upper-chest clavicular area, into an expansion that opens all bronchi. This practice can be deeply nourishing and feel incredibly transformative.

PARTICULARS AND PRECAUTIONS

- Cultivates focus, balance and gently invigorates.
- Expands often-neglected side/back areas of the lungs.
- Appropriate any time of day/evening.
- Utilized alone, in asana, and in life activities as a system balancer.
- Good in postures where spine is supported, and core engagement is not needed; avoid in vigorous asanas.
- Full Complete breath demands a relaxation of the stabilizing pelvic floor and lower abdominal muscles, so it is not appropriate for active asana or any body movement where spinal stabilization is needed.
- Full list of Immunity and Whole Health Benefits, page 44.

The tension of held, suppressed emotions is often present in the lower abdominal region and the area of the lungs, as well as the pit of the throat. One aspect of the transformational experience with this expansive breath is that held emotional tensions may be released. You may experience unexplained tears or laughter. This is normal and healthy. Allow for the release of this tension in those areas. Consider not suppressing any natural urges to release and trust the process of the body opening and healing.

Stabilize body, elongate spine, cultivating balance; sitting or reclined position can be used, although a Supta Baddha Konasana/Supported Bound Angle posture (described on page 208) can be an ideal position to fully support these openings.

- Inhale through the nose while calmly noting the length of the breath, creating a sustainable fullness.
- Guide the exhalation out the nostrils for the same length and quality.
- Focus on expanding the front, side, back of lower belly region, under the navel, with the inhalation.
- Relax the lower abdominal wall all the way down into the perineum or area between genital and anus. Inhale to expand and relax that area to a sustainable yet full capacity.
- Repeat three to six cycles,
- Adding Part II expansion, begin to build the fullness of the inhalation to include the lower abdominal cavity and add on a bit higher, by the bottom ribs, the mid-thoracic chest area which includes the lungs.
- Repeat three to six cycles.
- Adding Part III expansion, begin to build the fullness of the inhalation to include the lower abdominal cavity and mid-thoracic chest area, and now include the clavicular area that expands to the entire upper back and lower throat pit area.
- Create a fluidity of this three-part expansion, with no pauses.
- Repeat three to six cycles.
- Release, reset, and sit quietly, observing the effects of the practice.

UJJAYI PRANAYAMA
(OO-JAI-EE)
VICTORIOUS BREATH

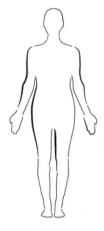 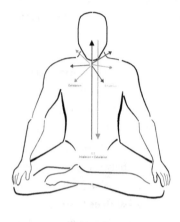

GROUNDING, FOCUS, GENTLY INVIGORATING, WARMS THE BODY

Often utilized while practicing asana, *ujjayi* breathing translates to "Victorious Breath" and is sometimes referred to as Ocean Breath, per the sound that is heard when it is practiced. Though modern-day teachings of this breath often compare it to the sound of Darth Vader, that strength of sound may be too harsh for the cardiovascular system as well as the vocal cords. Ideally, the practitioner or someone right next to them can hear the sound, but not an entire room.

PARTICULARS AND PRECAUTIONS

- Cultivates focus, endurance and gently invigorates.
- Massages and stimulates glands and vocal cords in the throat.
- Appropriate any time of day/evening; avoid directly before bedtime.
- Generally used with postures, especially the more vigorous dynamic series, to create heat in the body.
- Volume of breath loud enough for you, maybe some directly beside you, not entire room.
- Full list of Immunity and Whole Health Benefits, page 44.

Stabilize body, elongate spine, cultivating balance; sitting or reclined position can be used.

- Breathe through the nostrils creating balance of 1:1 or *sama vritti.*
- Create a slight constriction in the throat, creating a gentle oceanlike sound (tutorial below).
- Use gentle restriction, slowing the breath on both the inhalation and exhalation.
- This balanced breath can be utilized while doing postures, in combination with other breathing techniques, or while doing simple household tasks, as it cultivates a level of mastery and mindfulness.

CLEANING THE EYEGLASSES OR MIRROR EXERCISE
(Learning tool for ujjayi breathing)

Exercise on How to Create a Gentle Warming Constriction in the Throat Utilized in Ujjayi Breath:
Lift your dominant hand to just in front of your mouth, as if you are holding eyeglasses or a mirror. Open the mouth and create a heating moist exhalation breath on your hand. Do this a couple of times getting that constriction feeling clear in the body. Now close the lips and continue to make the heating exhalation breath. Nothing has changed other than the lips being closed, notice the gentle sound of the ocean that it creates. Now keep that same constriction, heating, and sound, and repeat with an inhale through the nose. Practice and repeat (avoid creating too much volume, just enough for you to hear and possibly the person beside you) this constriction and ocean sound, which is also called *ujjayi pranayama.*

VISAMA VRITTI PURAKA
(VEE-SAH-MA VREE-TEE POO-RAH-KAH)
UNEVEN INHALE BREATHING

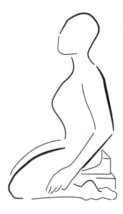 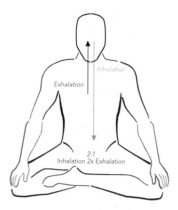

GENTLY INVIGORATING, CALM ALERT STATE, OPENS DIAPHRAGM/LUNGS

Use a 2:1 ratio to cultivate an inhalation twice as long as the exhalation. This increased inhalation creates a subtle balanced-energized feeling and mental clarity. This is a wonderful breath to do in midafternoon if you feel lazy or sleepy, in place of the afternoon sugar or caffeine snack!

PARTICULARS AND PRECAUTIONS

- Gentle awakening, concentration, endurance, and gently invigorating.
- Appropriate any time of day/evening; avoid directly before bedtime.
- Can be combined with ujjayi breathing for increased focus and invigoration.
- Cultivate the 2:1 ratio length without undue effort or strain.
- Full list of Immunity and Whole Health Benefits page 44.

Stabilize body, elongate spine, cultivating balance; sitting or reclined position can be used.

- Exhale the breath completely out.
- Inhale through the nose while calmly noting the length of the breath.
- Create a sustainable fullness in the inhalation.
- Exhale out the nostrils for only half of the length of the inhalation.
- Repeat and stabilize the cadence of the twice-as-long inhalation to exhalation.
- Start with the ratio of 6-count inhalation to a 3-count exhalation, build to 8:4 or possibly 10:5.
- Avoid strain caused by overextending the breaths.
- Release, reset, and sit quietly observing the effects of the practice.

SURYA BHEDANA
(SOO-REE-AH BED-AH-NA)
RIGHT NOSTRIL DOMINANCE BREATH

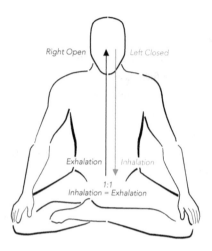

GENTLY INVIGORATING, FOCUS, OPENS RIGHT NOSTRIL, STIMULATES LEFT
HEMISPHERE OF BRAIN

Surya means sun, and this mindful solar breathing is a perfect energizing yet
stabilizing way to invigorate. When practiced with a steady repetition, it will
create that mental and physical clarity without jolting the system. I start my day
with a series of rounds of this breath and utilize it in the afternoons when I may
start to feel sluggish or dull. I am always amazed at the peaceful energized state
it creates. Note this is repetitive breathing through the right nostril only; there is
another surya pranayama that inhales through the right and out through the left
in repetition, which is also energizing and has a stronger effect on the system.
Integrate this foundational breathing before adding variations.

PARTICULARS AND PRECAUTIONS

- Gentle awakening, concentration, endurance, and gently invigorating.
- Right nostril stimulation increases left-brain (logical/linear) activity.
- Appropriate any time of day/evening; avoid directly before bedtime.

- Can be combined with ujjayi breathing for increased focus and invigoration.
- Cultivate the 1:1 or 2:1 ratio length without undue effort or strain.
- Full list of Immunity and Whole Health Benefits page 44.

HOW TO DO IT

Stabilize body, elongate spine, cultivating balance; sitting or reclined position can be used.

- Exhale the breath completely out.
- Close the left nostril with the dominant-hand middle finger, gentle pressure at the end of the cartilage.
- Keep that nostril closed during the entirety of breath repetitions.
- Inhale and exhale through the right nostril only, creating a sustainable expansive breath pattern.

The active dominant nostril is the one with more airflow and the passive nondominant one will have little to none. Oftentimes you can feel this dominance with the breath or with the index finger just at the nostril openings, and it can also be fun to check it out with a mirror. Placing a mirror just under the nostrils, gently breathe out, and one nostril will fog up the mirror much more than the other. Now, what's even more interesting and fun is noting what mental/emotional state you are in and seeing if it coincides with that dominant nostril! The right nostril aligns with the left or logical hemisphere of the brain, considered to be tied to the sympathetic nervous system, and the left nostril aligns with the right or creative/receptive hemisphere as well as the parasympathetic nervous system or rest/digest. If you feel mellow and relaxed, is the left nostril more active? If you feel very awake or even tense, is the right nostril dominant?

THYMUS GLAND TAPPING AND OM TONING

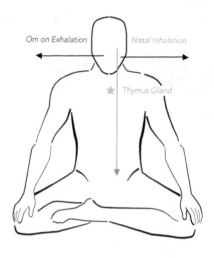

Om on Exhalation Nasal Inhalation

Thymus Gland

AWAKENING, GENTLY INVIGORATING, STIMULATE IMMUNE FUNCTION

Directly stimulate immune function with humming and tapping to create vibration and circulation of resources in and around the thymus gland. Synchronizing the breath, the sound vibration of OM, and tapping with intention is a total powerhouse of mind/body immunity-boosting! The thymus gland is a key player in the regulation of the immune system. As we age, it can atrophy, and by warming, vibrating, and circulating blood and oxygen to it, we give it a boost. OM is the vibration of universal harmony and is considered the most potent sound vibration or *mantra* available to us. On its own, it is a physical, mental, and emotional change agent. Consider practicing this every day, a minimum of three OMs per session, at least once and, on some days, multiple times throughout the day. It can be an easy, effective, and feel-good reset practice whenever needed.

PARTICULARS AND PRECAUTIONS

- Gently invigorating and directly stimulates immune function.
- Stimulates circulation in the thymus gland (main immune support gland).

- Increase blood, oxygen, and prana while decreasing stagnation, supporting detox.
- Appropriate any time of day/evening; avoid directly before bedtime.
- Steady yet gentle tapping, not enough to bruise, yet strong enough for stimulation.
- Cultivate sustainable vibration and tapping without undue effort or strain.
- Full list of Immunity and Whole Health Benefits page 44.

HOW TO DO IT

Stabilize body, elongate spine, cultivating balance; standing, sitting, or reclined position can be used.

- Exhale the breath completely out.
- Using the dominant-hand middle finger, identify the sternum bone, just under the jugular notch or throat pit area, and then drop down one inch below the sternum bone above the heart. This is the region around and above the thymus gland.
- Inhale deeply through the nose.
- Tap with the middle and ring finger pads below the sternum above the heart.
- Exhale on an OM vibration, toning on your exhalations as you tap above the thymus gland.
- This is pure sound vibration; there is no need to attempt to create pleasant tone, like singing.
- Envision a pure energy of healing as you tone and tap.
- Consider doing three rounds of toning tapping, three times each round, daily.

GYANA MUDRA
(GEE AHN A)
WISDOM HAND SEAL

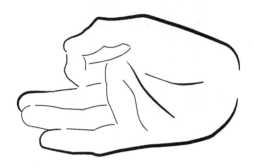

CLARITY, FOCUS, EXPANDS AWARENESS

Mudra is a seal or gesture that circulates pranic energy and invokes an experience of awareness within the body. It creates subtle neuronal connections within the conscious and subconscious to create healing and shift. It is body language, a subtle and powerful way of moving the mental, emotional body into a clear message to cultivate limbic resonance.

In this case, the *Gyana Mudra* is the wisdom seal, drawing awareness and life force through the body into the frontal lobe, the inner vision or third-eye center—the seat of wisdom. This *mudra* is a wholistic tool that enhances other breathing and meditations you may be practicing, amplifying the movement of life force. It adds an additional layer of subtle subconscious communications for the system and can be practiced alone or in conjunction with both postures and breathing exercises.

PARTICULARS AND PRECAUTIONS

- Enhances vital energy circulation to frontal lobe/third-eye center.
- Cultivates positive outcome, fortifying the RAS system in the brain (described page 41).

- Appropriate any time of day/evening.
- Steady yet gentle pressure in finger pads without undue effort or strain.

Stabilize body, elongate spine, cultivating balance; sitting or reclined position can be used.

- On both hands, press thumb pad and index finger pads gently yet firmly to touch, creating a loop.
- Relax remaining fingers on both hands and allow to rest naturally.
- Ease any tensions from the hand and reinforce the connection of the loop of thumb and index finger.
- Turn hands upward for inspiration and downward for grounding stabilization.
- Avoid unnecessary tension in the hands, elbows, shoulders, neck, and jaw while practicing.
- Become aware of any pulsations or tingling through the fingers and hands, as well as anywhere circulating through the body.
- Notice how you feel with the mudra and without the mudra.

CLARITY INTENTION SETTING MEDITATION

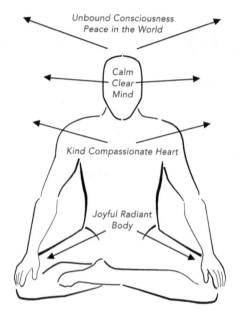

Unbound Consciousness
Peace in the World

Calm
Clear
Mind

Kind Compassionate Heart

Joyful Radiant
Body

SYSTEM RESET, INTENTION CULTIVATION, CREATES FEELING OF WELL-BEING

This simple yet potent focused awareness meditation was originally inspired by the stellar author/teacher Deepak Chopra. Its wholistic practicality had such an impact on me that I began to adapt and utilize it in many forms, including as a moving meditation as I went about my mundane household tasks to enhance them. The connection of intention and body is tangible and immediately effective. Simply having these intentions of Joyful Radiant Body, Loving Compassionate Heart, Calm Clear Mind and Unbound Consciousness/Peace in the World is enough to positively change your health, life, and beyond. Consider starting and ending the day with these intentions. As you become more familiar, it may become an easy reset for you in any moment of need.

- Creates a sense of well-being, relaxation, and whole-system harmony.
- Stimulates the relaxation and rest/digest response.
- Cultivates positive outcome, fortifying the reticular activating system.
- Utilize as a reset or efficient shifting whenever needed.
- Full list of Immunity and Whole Health Benefits page 44.

HOW TO DO IT

Stabilize body, elongate spine, cultivating balance; sitting or reclined position can be used.

- Create *Gyana Mudra/* Wisdom Hand Seal with both hands resting, the palms turned up, on the thighs.
- Bring awareness to the breath; feel the coolness of the air entering at the nasal openings.
- Observe the navel moving out as you inhale and in on the exhalation.
- Close the eyes, and inwardly follow the belly slowly moving out and in.
- Create an effortless balance of inhalation with exhalation or *sama vritti.*
- Recall the happiest, most joyful awareness or memory into your heart.
- Remember it and feel it in the whole body, as if permeating every cell of the body.
- Begin internally repeating the affirmation "Joyful Radiant Body."
- Allow it to go silent into an echo, continuing to feel the effects.
- Bring awareness into your heart.
- Feel your heart steady and spacious.
- Begin internally repeating the affirmation "Loving Compassionate Heart."
- Allow it to go silent into an echo, continuing to feel the effects.
- Bring awareness between the eyebrows or to the third-eye center.
- Feel your mind steady and spacious.
- Begin internally repeating the affirmation "Calm Clear Mind."
- Allow it to go silent into an echo, continuing to feel the effects.

- Move your awareness beyond your physical body, connecting to the vast universe in and around you.
- Feel the essence in and around you steady and spacious.
- Begin internal repeating the affirmation "Unbound Consciousness, Peace in the World."
- Allow it to go silent into an echo, continuing to feel the effects.
- Draw into your body and simply be aware.
- Become aware of your heartbeat.
- Become aware of the pulse of life in your heart.
- Being aware is connection to your own highest intelligence.
- Become aware of the pulse of life between your thumb pad and index finger pad on both hands.
- Trace that pulse from your hands up the forearms, the shoulders, back into the heart, and throughout the entire body.
- Gently breathe into the body with this whole-being clarity and awareness.
- Consider reclining on to the back to rest and reset in Shavasana/ Corpse Pose page 214.

CHAPTER 4

SEQUENCES FOR CLARITY

If the poses on their own are like individual foods as a snack, putting them all together in a sequence creates an entire meal. There are as many sequence possibilities as there are recipes for delicious meals. Those below are simply a jumping-off point, and I hope that one day you are cooking up a storm, creating many different sequences with the poses and breathing exercises in the previous chapters and beyond.

In this chapter, I share four foundational, entry-level meals that are short and easy to incorporate every day.

You can do the Daily Mini Sequence either standing or sitting, and for those who are at a desk working much of the day, I recommend doing both! Start with doing this three-minute practice, incorporate it into your life both morning and afternoon, and eventually you can add postures from Chapter 2 into it to grow it as you go.

The following sequences are in this order

1. Three-Minute Daily Essential Mini Sequence (Standing Version)
2. Three-Minute Daily Essential Mini Sequence (Seated Version)
3. Eight-Minute Clarity Practice Sequence
4. Clarity Breathing Sequence

1
THREE-MINUTE DAILY ESSENTIAL MINI
SEQUENCE (STANDING VERSION)

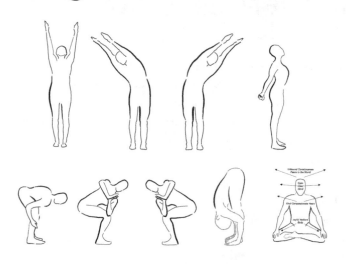

#2
THREE-MINUTE DAILY ESSENTIAL MINI
SEQUENCE (SEATED VERSION)

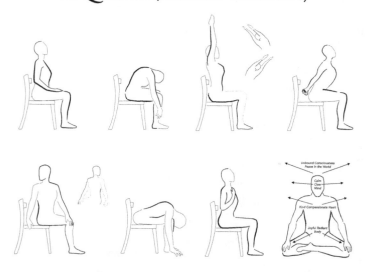

#3
EIGHT-MINUTE CLARITY PRACTICE SEQUENCE

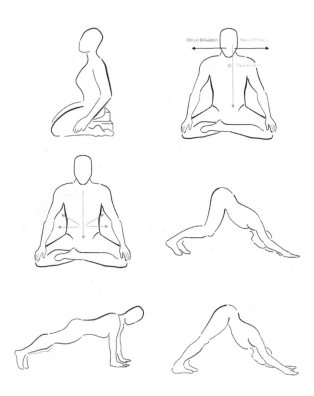

→

Transition to standing

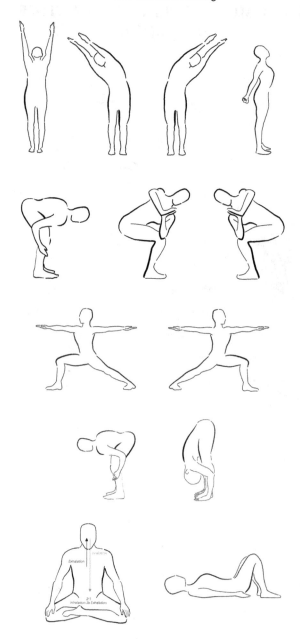

#4
CLARITY BREATHING SEQUENCE

Do breathing either reclined or upright.

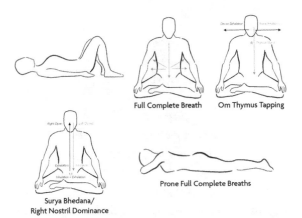

Full Complete Breath   Om Thymus Tapping

Surya Bhedana/
Right Nostril Dominance

Prone Full Complete Breaths

Do Expansive 3 Part Breaths either reclined or upright.

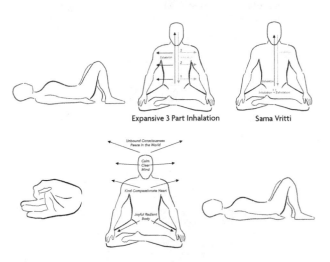

Expansive 3 Part Inhalation   Sama Vritti

"ONLY ONE THING? DO THIS."

Chapter 1

Get clear on what is essential to you and align your actions/practices/ habits to that.

Chapter 2

Track your daily physical patterns to discover imbalances. Move the spine in all directions *every day*.

Chapter 3

Breathe deeply through the nose fully expanding the front, sides and back of the lower abdomen throughout the day.

Chapter 4

Three-Minute Daily Essential Mini Sequence (Seated Version)

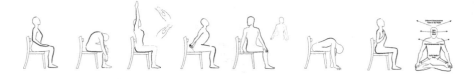

"Joyful Radiant Body
Kind Compassionate Heart
Calm Clear Mind
Unbound Consciousness, Peace in the World"

PART II

DETOXIFICATION

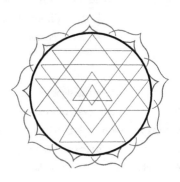

CLEARING TO MAKE SPACE

When we are stressed out, it weakens our immune system. De-stressing ourselves is the number-one thing we can do to boost our immunity.

Ahead in Chapter 6, we will explore how stress and toxins stagnate the body and the importance of spinal rotation to massage the abdominal cavity and detox the lymphatic channels of the body. In Chapter 7, we will learn how to clean out the lungs of stale air as well as clearing out stuck emotions that can drain us of our peace and vitality. Here we will investigate what may be stressing us out or creating a stress overload response and exploring the practices to reduce those stressors and lighten our load.

Stress can come in many forms, some obvious, some not. Stressors such as poor air quality, big life events, working long hours, lack of sleep, worrying, accumulation of daily hassles, poor diet, and even dehydration can stress us out and lower our immune function.

Our job is to become more sensitive to the signs of too much stress and cues of toxin overload. We function on many levels of awareness, and I am referring to multisystem signals such as sensations, pains, mental-emotional states of being, and intuitive understandings. As we detox and simplify, we unify all the parts of awareness and ideally catch the signals of imbalance before we go into true suffering or dis-ease.

"Let go or be dragged." A voice woke me up in the middle of the night. I had been feeling crappy for a while. It wasn't just one thing; it was a lot of things, as I was holding on to so much and so stressed out. I was tired yet wired and tense. My stomach was upset and burning after meals. My skin was broken out and I had an itchy rash on my arm. In truth, it was nothing compared to the chronic hives that were driving me crazy. Maybe it was the sinus meds, as my nose had been stuffed up for days. I'd just been so tired I couldn't think straight. It was nothing a mocha latte couldn't fix. I was in a chronic stress overdrive response here. Does any of this sound familiar to you?

CHRONIC STRESS OVERDRIVE RESPONSE

Many of us are in a chronic stress overload, and our sympathetic nervous system is in an overdrive response, meaning it is in a constant cycle of fight-or-flight without end. When we are in a chronic stress response, we may experience anxiety, tension, cardiovascular issues, high blood pressure, high blood sugar, insulin resistance, cortisol overload, sleep problems, brain fog, emotional reactivity, digestive issues, food sensitivities, acne, rashes, increased abdominal fat, and *suppressed immune function*. (I know we could add more to this list!) Our culture thrives on messages of ignoring pain and pushing for results. No pain no gain, take a pill and get over it.

This go-go-go can take our vital resources away from our longevity functions supported by the parasympathetic nervous system or rest/digest response. The issue comes from the fact that the "fight or flight" mode is designed for a quick burst of adrenaline to give us short-lived strength and speed to either fight or flee the tiger. It is not designed to fight or flee the tiger in an eighty-year nonstop war, just an eight-minute battle. It makes perfect sense that, if we were stuck in chronic battle response, we would become sick and drained. It is also noteworthy to mention that in our current world, the tiger comes in many perceived forms and can be triggered with a simple ding chime from your email app. We are inundated with triggers in our day and once we begin to see that clearly, we can begin to address it, one stressor at a time.

PAY ATTENTION TO THE CUES

When "Let go or be dragged" shook me out of my fitful sleep, I had been completely ignoring my body's cues, and now my intuitive wisdom was taking over. I was awake, stunned, and processing with unmistakable clarity that it was time for me to take care of my business—the business of de-stressing my life, clearing my body and shifting harmful habits and choices that were hurting me. I had been pushing, ignoring warning signals physically and emotionally, and I could no longer deny it was time to make a change.

This was a startling turning point in my life, my body screaming at me, and my inner voice booming. It's one that I now call upon often to reinspire me to continue the work to de-stress my life and make better choices. I translate the inner voice saying to me," Hey, pay attention, stop killing yourself and clean up your act!" There were things I was refusing to acknowledge in my life that were hurting me, and many of them were my own doing. I was experiencing stressors from every angle; diet, lack of sleep, work, relationships, and suppressed emotions, you name it, my body and nervous system were simply overloaded.

ACKNOWLEDGMENT WILL CALM THE BODY DOWN AND BEGIN THE HEALING PROCESS

As Dr. Daniel Siegal, a psychiatrist renowned for his work with brain science, mindfulness, and well-being, coined the phrase," Name it to tame it." Naming the underlying emotion or stress of a situation will help the nervous system calm down and come out of the reactive stress response. When we are stressed and experiencing overload, this tool guides us to pull back from the response and name the cause with emotion attached that is overloading us.

For example, the ping of a work text message may trigger the fight-or-flight response because, if we don't answer it soon enough, we may be perceived as slacking off, which could lead to losing our jobs, which brings up fear. It is the tiger that is chasing us. We often rationalize that response to suppress it. It sits in the subconscious, having an accumulative effect of sapping our vitality and shifting energy away from our longevity functions, like our immune system. It creates a baseline of chronic stress.

Taking a pause and stepping back to name it will create the space for shifting the nervous system out of the stress response into the clearer thinking of the rest/digest mode.

When you acknowledge it: "I feel fear when I hear the ping sound from my phone, it freaks me out like I am going to lose my job." There may be a flood of relief and compassion. It is an Aha! moment that frees you from this unconscious stress cycle. It tames the response and creates a system homeostasis for you to help yourself. Our yoga practice cultivates that mindfulness and ability to pause, feel, create space from the experience, to unhook from the stress cycle and redirect ourselves to compassion and healing connection.

TAKING INVENTORY CREATES CLARITY AND CALMNESS

The first step for me, after the night of receiving that inner wakeup call, was to begin taking an honest inventory of where I was overloaded. I created time to sit in quiet, wrapped in my favorite blanket with my journal, and to take inventory of where I was hurting or challenged. It helped to create calm for myself and distance from the reactivity of it to see it more clearly. From that calm distance, I named what was underlying each area. That naming it helped my whole system relax and gave me greater understanding to then choose mindful next steps to realign those areas of my life.

SUPPRESS IT AND IT WILL GET WORSE

Our job is to create a clarity in the mind and body so we can be more sensitive to the cues and wisdom messages we are receiving. The yogic practices train us to feel the cue and then mindfully respond. Cultivating the first tenet of the yoga practice (first of the eight limbs), *ahimsa*/non-harm, so that we can do no harm to our body and respond accordingly to the second tenet, *satya*/truthfulness.

The poses are an excellent arena to learn to listen to the physical as well as emotional cues. As we pause and tune into the body and breath, we break the cycle of ignoring and can really tap into what we are being called to address. It is this perfect opportunity to get a sense of what is needed in a safe separate moment, away from regular bustle of life.

INVENTORY TO HELP US LISTEN TO THE CUES OF IMBALANCE

This aspect of self-study is the foundation of whole health and a yoga practice. It is the important foundation that will make all the actions of caretaking more potent. It may not feel fun to look at harmful habits, areas of life that aren't working, and our stressors, yet it is essential to supporting whole health and happiness.

Let's take inventory and compassionately explore the inquiries below. Question, feel, contemplate, and consider writing down your unedited responses. Allow it to be messy, and kindly give yourself room to be imperfect.

- What is *in the way* of you living what is essential to you, or what are *the main obstacles?*
- What are the stressors in your life that are draining you of your vitality and joy?
- What area of life or situation are you suppressing or ignoring?
- What choices consciously or unconsciously are you making that are harming you?
- Are there seemingly minor issues that you may be ignoring?
- What is your inner wisdom trying to tell you?
- Where do you feel that in your body?
- How does stress show up for you physically?
- How does stress show up for you mentally?
- How does stress show up for you emotionally?
- What is it time for you to do or change?

Gently coax out what may be under the surface and bring it into the light of conscious awareness. In this way, we air it out and name it to tame it. When it is in the light, we can take clear steps to acknowledge, hear, and transform to heal. When we have clarity, then we can take the steps needed to move forward. It is that simple.

DEEPER INVENTORY OF TENDENCIES AND DAILY HABITS

Our habits become us. Not all habits are bad, in fact many habits are excellent and help us thrive. It is our job to identify which habits need to go and which we will amplify to do even greater good for our lives.

Years ago, a wise friend said to me in passing, "Only repeat what you want to continue." Those words forever echo with me. Exactly! Because repetition and its accumulative effect is powerful, we only want to repeat what we want to continue. Then why the heck do we keep repeating what we don't want?

Let's explore these inquiries and look at what we are repeating:

- What are you repeating that is helpful for you?
- *Consider making a list starting with the most mundane, for example: wash my face before bedtime.*
- What are you repeating that is harmful to you?
- Why do you repeat the habits that are harmful?
- What need does it fulfill?

Where is there an opportunity to replace a harmful habit with a helpful one to support that need?

In my mid-twenties, living in Los Angeles, sitting in (a lot of) traffic in my little green Honda Civic, I listened to many hours of the talks of educator Stephen Covey, the author of *The 7 Habits of Highly Effective People*, and he said, "We become what we repeatedly do." It was then that I started to really look at my daily habits and create conscious changes.

The funny thing about habits is that, once we do something one time, it becomes much easier to do it a second time. It is the way our brain creates neuro-connections to reduce the amount of energy we are expending throughout the day. Also interesting is that, once the brain makes that connection or pathway for that habit, it never goes away. In this way, you can never actually break a bad habit, yet you can create a whole new one, placing your energy into the new habit as the old one fades away in the background.

The good news is that many of the practices in this book may be totally new to you, but once you do them one time, it will be easier for you to do them again and again...and to make a lifetime healthy habit. And my hope is that, as you identify the harmful habits in your life, you will be able to begin the journey of replacing them with something helpful, and therefore making the harmful habits obsolete and eliminating them.

Ignored symptoms and cues of imbalance, harmful habits, and toxic self-talk are all contributors to being stressed out and the weakening of immune function. James Clear, author of the book *Atomic Habits*, writes, "A lack of self-awareness is poison. Reflection and review is the antidote."

The last area of review and reflection may be the trickiest and yet most powerfully revealing. Intentionally listen to yourself (both to what you say out loud and to your internal dialogue) to get a window into greater truth and insight into your inner stress.

This is important, as what is undermining our immunity and our whole health is often hidden deep in our subconscious. It is programming and thoughts that are so subtle, and often so familiar, we don't recognize them. These very subtle whispers in our mind create stress. That undercurrent of stress when not named will go untamed and undermine the healing work we are attempting on the surface. This is root work to begin to expose what is underneath the more obvious system.

Consider exploring these and taking special care when you are in conversation throughout your days.

What do you say about yourself to other people?
What may that reveal?

What do you say about yourself to yourself?
What may that reveal?

By bringing this forward in your awareness, how can you shift to be kinder and more supportive to yourself?

Begin to look for patterns in your answers within the previous inquiries. Do you see any recurring themes in what you may be ignoring or avoiding? What feelings may be being suppressed? What needs or cues are being ignored? In what areas of your body do you feel that stress? Where is there a need for attention? Is it your physical body, your emotional life, your mental stress, or is it all of it needing to be in greater alignment to your wisest inner self? Hopefully that helps guide you to clarity to choose one area to give your attention to.

What are you ready to clear to make room for greater health, joy, and abundance?

Implement one micro habit to support de-stressing your body and mind.
Say it out loud. Write it down. Do a mental rehearsal for it each day until it is anchored and effortless.

Create a specific plan of action for how you will implement this new helpful habit. After what will you do it, for how long, and right before what next action?

Example: In the evening, right after I brush my teeth and put my toothbrush in the closet, I will _____
(new helpful habit) for three minutes and then take my shower.

If you are not sure exactly what to implement, hint: any of the practices offered so far could be an excellent choice!

Keep it simple and choose one that feels good so you *want to continue it*. Consider incorporating this new habit in an ongoing way to create consistency. Sometimes the things that are draining us may feel like a mountain. We can move them one pebble, one small choice at a time. We can also shift how we think about them and our relationship to them. With each inquiry, practice, and breath, we get clearer and make healing progress.

The wonderful news is that, just by having done the exploration of this chapter, you have already begun the shift of healing. You are already more aware, and that in itself will have cleared some of these tendencies and created greater alignment. You are already better off!

CHAPTER 6

ASANA FOR DETOXIFICATION

Simply put: good stuff in and bad stuff out. Equal and opposite to create balance. The poses in this chapter are important to help move metabolic waste out of the system as well as aid in circulation through the entire body. We create space for nourishment and healing by clearing out the waste and toxins.

MOVEMENT AND SPINAL ROTATION FOR DETOXIFICATION

By the use of leg activation, core engagement, and twisting the upper back, we compress and then release the abdominal cavity. This positively affects the nervous, pulmonary, digestive, and cardiovascular systems, and greatly aids in spinal health. When we rotate the spine, we lubricate the joints, refresh the spinal fluid, and renew the discs which serve as shock absorbers, supporting spinal health and movement as well as the stability of the spine. We are as young and healthy as the spinal column, the central pillar of structural support as well as support of cerebral grey matter that communicates with the rest of the body.

KEY TO SAFE SPINAL ROTATION

A key principle of safety for twisting the spine is to lengthen the spine first before rotating, drawing the sternum up away from the base to make room along the intervertebral discs, so when the twisting happens, there is no undue stress on the discs, which can cause injury. The intervertebral discs are jelly-donut-like shock absorbers in the spine. Imagine that fresh, fragrant, just-baked jelly donut from your favorite bakery. If you push on the donut with too much force, the jelly comes out. Your spinal discs are similar, if there is too much gravitational pressure on the discs while you rotate, they are at risk for bulging or herniation. When we lengthen through the spine, we create room for the discs to plump up. Once they plump up a bit, then we mindfully twist the spine on the axis of the center (not swiveling or swaying out to the side) to rinse and soak the discs. We squeeze out the old fluid and, when we return to neutral, flood the disc with fresh synovial fluid. That action reminds me of squeezing out a water-filled sponge as we wring the discs out and fill them back up for optimum health.

MASSAGE THE ABDOMINAL CAVITY TO ELIMINATE WASTE

When we don't properly eliminate waste, we get sick. Twisting supports proper elimination and a healthy gastrointestinal tract, which is why the next series of poses will help create space in the spine and room for the internal organs, and then twist out toxins, so when the body comes back to neutral, it will be renewed. The massaging pressure on the internal organs from rotation and spinal movements also aids in clearing the lungs of stale air as well as aiding lymphatic drainage.

AIDING LYMPHATIC CIRCULATION A DETOXIFICATION AND IMMUNITY BOOST

Lymph nodes are part of the immune system and filter invaders like virus and toxins through lymphatic fluid. The channels of fluid and clusters of small bean sized nodules are found throughout the body, and the postural practice helps circulate out the toxins. The lymph nodes are checkpoints in the groin, armpits, throat, neck, and head. They hold white blood cells that directly attack virus, bacteria, and abnormal cells, and detains them. The lymph can swell and become overloaded with toxin and debris. Yoga postures and breathing techniques can help clear that debris by stimulating circulation of the lymphatic fluid and directly aid immune function.

Remembering your intention as clarity brings energy to your actions.

Connecting back into your why, weaving essential intentions into your actions, creates a potent energy of follow-through. Whether you call it inspiration, discipline, or pranic energy, it is the "it" aspect that creates transformation.

Continue to breathe slowly and intentionally through the nostrils and with the visualization or mental rehearsal of what you want, and consciously train the reticular activating system, that guidance system for creating successful transformation, before you do each pose. Keep it simple, and in the beginning, possibly say it out loud. It doesn't need to take long, just a simple flash of your mental rehearsal and it will support your practice. Again, even though you are clearing out here with detox practices, continue to direct the mind to a dress rehearsal of what you want, not what you don't want.

IMMUNITY BENEFITS FOR THE FOLLOWING DETOXIFICATION POSTURES

- Increases oxygen/blood circulation, decreases stagnation and toxins.
- Aids in digestion, breathing, and cardiovascular, brain, and glandular function.
- Increases spinal mobility and aids elimination (twist variations).
- Supports expansion of the diaphragm and the lungs.
- Decreases inflammation and aids in lymphatic drainage.
- Supports the rest/digest response of parasympathetic nervous system.
- Supports mental/emotional outlook, releasing endorphins, serotonin, and dopamine.
- Increases stamina, endurance, and resilience.
- Creates feelings of release, freedom, focus, and courage.
- Activates vital energy (pranic) lines through the entire body.

POSES FOR DETOXIFICATION

MALASANA
(MA-LAH-SAH-NA)
SQUAT POSE

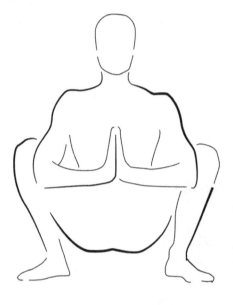

OPENING, ENERGIZING, HELPS ELIMINATION

Also known as defecation pose, this is an important posture for strengthening the ability to eliminate and clear physically as well as emotionally. This practicing of bearing down, yet lifting up strength and stability from the earth, can be an ideal birthing position for a healthy unmedicated birth. To create balance in the emptying-out movement, stabilizing of the pelvic floor is also needed in balanced opposition, so even though it may seem like we are dropping down, we are in truth activating a lift up through the core as we squat down. If the depth of the squat is unsustainable for your body, sit lifted on blocks, on the edge of a stable chair, or in a higher lifted position. What are you clearing to make room for what you are cultivating or birthing into your life?

STRETCHES (CREATING SPACE)

- Stretches the feet, calves, legs, hips, buttocks, and low back.
- Opens pelvis and pelvic outlet, creating space for abdominal organs.

STRENGTHENS (CREATING STEADINESS)

- Strengthens legs, buttocks, pelvic floor, spinal column.
- Builds stamina and balance.
- Strengthens digestion, elimination, and the reproductive organs.

PARTICULARS AND PRECAUTIONS

- Can be cooling or heating depending on practitioner.
- Appropriate any time of day or evening.
- Supports downward movement of waste for detoxification.
- Anchor heels on floor or with a blanket folded underneath to take pressure off the knees.
- Sit on two blocks or a sturdy chair, supporting the sitting bones to reduce strain.
- Avoid if knee issues, sciatica, uterine prolapse, hemorrhoids, high blood pressure, acute varicose veins.

Full list of Immunity and Whole Health Benefits, page 113.

HOW TO DO IT

Breathe, connect with intention, and visualize pose before doing.

- Start from Mountain Pose.
- Align feet slightly wider than hip-width, turn thighs out in external rotation.
- Bending the knees, align knees and feet in the same plane, draw the weight of the body into the heels.

- Lowering the hips and body as low as is sustainable, buttocks hovering over the heels of the feet.
- Root through the heels and lift up through the pelvic floor.
- Press palms together at the chest as in prayer mudra, pressing the heels of the hands together, invigorating both palms and wrists and helping the chest to expand.
- Lifting from the pelvic, core, spinal column, sternum, chest, and head.
- Align the chin parallel to the floor while holding the gaze straight ahead.
- Root into the feet and keeping the pelvic floor steady, as you learned with exercise on page 47.
- Inhale rebound through the body, lift chest, creating a clear intention of creating vitality and inspiration. Stay as long as sustainable, creating space in the abdominal cavity.
- Return to Mountain Pose or release into Child's Pose.

A *mala* in Sanskrit is a vehicle for eliminating impurities. This pose helps move out digestive and metabolic waste from the body, supporting the movement of the *apana vayu* of the pranic system.

PRASARITA PADOTTANASANA
(PRAS-A-REETA PAH-DOH-TAH-NAH-SA-NA)
WIDE LEG FORWARD FOLD

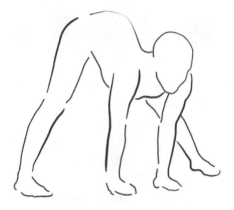

CALMING, COOLING, MASSAGES ABDOMEN, STRETCHES BACK OF THE LEGS

This pose can create delicious traction for the neck and spine, working with gravity to make space in the intervertebral discs (those jelly-donut shock absorbers in the spine). A misconception is that the goal of the posture is to get the top of the head on the floor. Although this can be utilized if the spine is completely long in its natural curves, for most bodies, this attempt will create unhealthy rounding of the spine and reduce the benefits of the posture. Focus on lengthening the front torso from pubis to the crown of the head and hinging from the hips, keeping that length the entire process maximizes the gravitational pull to create steady spaciousness.

STRETCHES (CREATING SPACE)

- Back of legs, hips, buttocks, spine creates traction for the spinal column
- Massage internal organs and abdomen

STRENGTHENS (CREATING STEADINESS)

- Outer ankles and legs
- Supports a feeling of stability and calmness

PARTICULARS AND PRECAUTIONS

- Cools and calms the body.
- Increases posterior lung expansion and air circulation.
- Appropriate any time of day/evening.
- Cultivates inversion benefits of circulating blood to heart.
- Can be practiced between other poses to calm and reset the system.
- Bend the knees if any strain in the low back, or micro bend knees for hyperextension.
- Place hands on block or on thighs for stability and to relieve the low back.
- Avoid if spinal disc issues or sciatic pain, eye issues, reflux, acute low blood pressure.
- Full list of Immunity and Whole Health Benefits, page 113.

HOW TO DO IT

Breathe, connect with intention, and visualize pose before doing.

- Start from Mountain Pose.
- Step the feet out a leg's distance apart with feet parallel to each other.
- Root the mound of the big toes as you activate the outer ankles in and up, avoiding sickling of ankles.
- Rooting feet and rebounding up the legs and base of the spine, through the center line of the body, drawing up through the arms to the fingertips, up into a wide V, inspired lift.
- Begin to fold, bend the knees to hinge from the hips, descend with a long spine, avoiding rounding.
- Lengthen the front of the torso as you fold, bending knees to keep pressure out of the low back.

- Steady the fold by engaging the legs and lowering the hands on the floor, directly under the shoulders, or onto something higher (seat of a chair or yoga blocks) if the spine is rounding.
- Stack the hips aligned over the heels with the weight of the body slightly forward.
- Breathe evenly and continue these actions as you lengthen through the legs, deepening the stretch to the back of the legs and front of the spine.
- Transition into the following Twisted Forward Fold.

PARVRITTA PRASARITA PADOTTANASANA
(PAR-VREE-TAH)
TWISTED WIDE LEG FORWARD FOLD

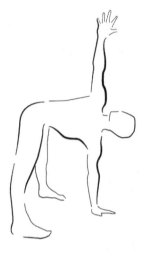

CALMING, DETOXIFYING, SUPPORTS FOCUS, STRETCHES BACK OF THE LEGS

HOW TO DO IT

Breathe, connect with intention, and visualize pose before doing.

- Starting in Wide Leg Forward Fold.
- Align hands under the shoulders, lift the chest toward parallel to the floor.
- Bring left hand to left hip in preparation to twist the chest to the left for a spinal twist.
- Use the left hand to apply gentle pressure, stabilizing the hip from excessive twisting or elevating.
- Inhale, lengthen the spine, drawing the upper back in, opening the chest.
- Engage the low belly to twist the chest open to the left side and, if stable, use the bottom arm for leverage.

- Stack the shoulders and reach through the upper arm.
- If the neck feels tight, keep the top arm down and hand on the outer hip.
- Inhale, lengthen spine; exhale, deepen the twist from belly into upper back.
- Return to center, stabilize, and then proceed to do the other side; equal time/quality.
- Preparing to exit the pose, place hands on the frontal hip bones, bend the knees, firm the thighs and belly in as you lift from the chest to come halfway upright; stabilize before coming all the way to stand.
- Return to Mountain Pose and consider adding a Sun Stretch Series before proceeding to Lunge Pose.

ANJANAYASANA
(AHN-JA-NAY-AH-SA-NA)
LUNGE POSE

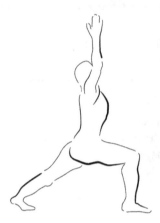

ENERGIZING, CLEARING, COURAGE, AND STAMINA-BUILDING

This asymmetric strength-building standing posture works the body in opposition to come to balance. We must work the polarities of the legs to bring the torso into supported length and invigoration. As it works the polarities of the physical body, it also works the mental and energetic opposites within our system. It is all about the legs or foundation of the pose here. When our legs or roots are strong, then the spine will be supported. When the spine or trunk is supported, we create far-reaching, powerful branches and sweet fruits of creation.

STRETCHES (CREATING SPACE)

- Stretches the front of back leg, hip, lower abdomen, torso, spine, chest, shoulders.
- Creates space in lower back, relieving back pain.

STRENGTHENS (CREATING STEADINESS)

- Strengthens feet, legs, buttocks, spine, core, lungs, heart, shoulders.
- Supports a feeling of focus, stability, and stamina.

- Creates heat in the body.
- Appropriate any time; avoid before bedtime.
- Avoid knee injury by keeping the knee stacked over the ankle and pointed straight ahead.
- Press back heel to a wall to energize the legs; utilize chair for balance.
- Avoid if acute low back or knee problems, extreme frailty; if high blood pressure, keep hands on the hips.
- Full list of Immunity and Whole Health Benefits, page 113.

HOW TO DO IT

Breathe, connect with intention, and visualize pose before doing.

- Start in Mountain or Chair Pose with feet hip-width apart and parallel to each other.
- Step the left foot back about a leg's distance apart from the front foot.
- Align the front right leg knee directly over the ankle and in line with the second toe of the foot.
- Engage the legs toward the midline, and firm the belly muscles to stabilize the opposition of the legs.
- Lengthen up through side waist so the torso is even on all sides.
- Reach the arms up in an inspired lift to create space in the lungs and upper body.
- Breathe ujjayi breaths and hold five to eight cycles of breath, or what is sustainable without strain.
- Bring hands to hips, engage the core muscles, shift weight more into the front foot to step up to reset.
- Return to center, stabilize, and then proceed to do the other side; equal time/quality.
- Return to Mountain or Chair Pose to reset, then proceed to the Lunge Twist.

PARVITTA ANJANAYASANA
TWISTED LUNGE POSE

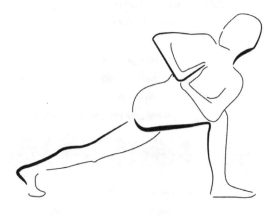

ENERGIZING, DETOXIFYING, COURAGE, AND STAMINA-BUILDING

Breathe, connect with intention, and visualize pose before doing.

- Start in Mountain or Chair Pose with feet hip-width apart and parallel to each other.
- Step the left foot back about a leg's distance apart from the front foot.
- Reach the arms up in an inspired lift to create space in the lungs and upper body.
- Bring palms together at the chest, preparing to twist the belly and upper back.
- Exhale, engage core muscles; draw the navel toward the spine and turn the chest in toward the leg.
- Utilize left hand or elbow on the outside of the left thigh for leverage (or block).
- Stabilize the legs and hips and focus the twist in the upper back.
- Inhale, lengthen through the spine; exhale, deepen the twist.

- Allow head to go along for the ride and follow the rotation led by the chest.
- Breathe ujjayi breaths and hold five to eight cycles of breath, or what is sustainable without strain.
- Bring hands to hips, engage the core muscles, shift weight more into the front foot to step up to reset.
- Return to center, stabilize, and then proceed to do the other side; equal time/quality.
- Return to Mountain or Chair Pose to reset; consider adding a Sun Stretch Series before lowering to the floor for Locust Pose.

SALABHASANA
(SHAHL-AH-BAHS-AH-NA)
LOCUST POSE

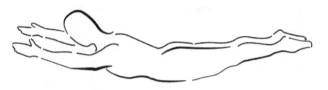

GENTLY ENERGIZING, CLEARING, SPINAL STRENGTHENING

Some backbends can energize the system, others strengthen. This strengthening and gentle opening backbend is wonderful to deepen determination, provide abdominal massage for the internal organs, and stabilize the spine. It is especially supportive to spinal health when the core muscles are properly engaged and the legs are in a neutral and active position, creating length in the low back. Whether a beginner or more advanced asana practitioner, incorporate this posture into your asana practice.

STRETCHES (CREATING SPACE)

- Stretches legs, abdomen, spine, chest, shoulders, entire front body.

STRENGTHENS (CREATING STEADINESS)

- Strengthens legs, spine, core, back, shoulders, entire back body.
- Builds stamina, stability, and focus.

PARTICULARS AND PRECAUTIONS

- Creates gentle heat in the body.
- Appropriate any time; avoid before bedtime.
- Cultivate length of spine versus high lift of torso and legs.
- Add block between the thighs as on page 47 to support core and spinal column.

- Keep arms by the side if shoulder, neck, high blood pressure issues.
- Keep feet on floor, legs down, if low back issues (half locust).
- Avoid if abdominal, spinal disc issues (anteriorly herniated), acute high blood pressure.
- Full list of Immunity and Whole Health Benefits, page 113.

Pause to practice full and complete belly breaths here, expanding the posterior lung capacity by pushing the navel into the floor while inhaling. Utilize any opportunity on the belly to integrate this lung-strengthening and nervous-system-soothing breathing.

HOW TO DO IT

Breathe, connect with intention, and visualize pose before doing.

- Start prone on the belly, forehead down, arms by the side, with feet hip-width and parallel to each other.
- Reach the arms forward along the head, activate the core to stabilize the upper back and spine.
- Lengthen through the legs and press the tops of the feet down to begin.
- Stabilize spine and stretch through body in opposite directions, eventually lifting legs, chest, and arms.
- Cultivate spinal and low back length over leg/arm lift.
- Repeat up to three times, then rest with one ear down to floor, then progress to alternate arm and leg variation.

VARIATION SALABHASANA
LOCUST POSE ALTERNATE ARM/LEG LIFT

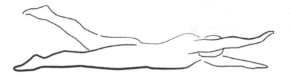

BALANCING, SPINAL STRENGTHENING, ENHANCES COGNITIVE FUNCTION

HOW TO DO IT

Breathe, connect with intention, and visualize pose before doing.

- Start prone on the belly, forehead down, arms reaching forward, feet hip-width, parallel to each other.
- Lift right arm and opposite side left leg, beginning dynamic lifts.
- Inhale lift, exhale lower.
- Inhale, lift left arm and (opposite side) right leg, cultivating more spinal length then arm/leg lift.
- Stabilize the spine and stretch through body in opposite directions as you alternate sides.
- Repeat complete rounds, up to three times, then rest with one ear down to floor, then proceed to C-Clasp Variation.

Alternating the arms and legs benefits core strength and stability as well as enhancing cognitive function as it activates both hemispheres of the brain, bringing system balance. The actions also stimulate and balance polar *pranic* energies equated to solar- and lunar-quality energies, bringing polarities to harmony.

VARIATION SALABHASANA
LOCUST POSE WITH A C-CLASP (ARMS BEHIND BACK)

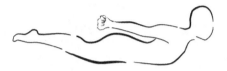

ENERGIZING, CLEARING, SPINAL STRENGTHENING

HOW TO DO IT

Breathe, connect with intention, and visualize pose before doing.

- Start prone on the belly, forehead down, arms by the side, with feet hip-width and parallel to each other.
- Reach the arms behind the back, activate the core to stabilize the upper back and spine.
- Lengthen through the legs and press the tops of the feet down to begin.
- Lengthen through the entire torso and arms to clasp hands together; link thumbs, use a yoga strap, or simply reach them back actively behind you.
- Inhale to stretch body open, exhale and firm the core to stabilize the spine.
- Breathe for up to five breath cycles.
- Release body and turn the head to one side.
- Either repeat pose or proceed to transition into Bow Pose.

Purpose of arms behind body is to help the upper back move in and chest to open, aiding in breath expansion, and counters habitual rounding of the upper back. Work to straighten the elbows as well as keeping the wrists straight to leverage the upper back in. As mentioned in description, you can do this with a thumb clasp, strap, or simple hands separated and active stretching. All are effective. Avoid jutting the chin forward, and direct length in all four sides of the neck while lengthening back through the rest of the body.

DHANURASANA
(DAWN-YUR-AH-SAH-NAH)
BOW POSE

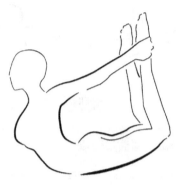

CLEARING, ENERGIZING, COURAGE BUILDING, CULTIVATES
BREATH EXPANSION

A quintessential freedom posture that you may have practiced in elementary school. I see you grinning with one of your front teeth missing—the opening up of hopeful possibility in this energizing and clearing backbend. The only difference from when you were eight years old is the wisdom to focus on containing and directing the pure life force by keeping the thighs together and hip-width apart. It will send arrow-like clarity through your spine and system as well as protect the low back. If that is not sustainable or is a strain, repeat Locust Pose with a C-Clasp (hands behind the back).

STRETCHES (CREATING SPACE)

- Stretches legs, abdomen, spine, chest, lungs, heart, shoulders, entire front body.

STRENGTHENS (CREATING STEADINESS)

- Strengthens legs, buttocks, spine, core, back, shoulders, entire back body.
- Builds energy, courage, and stamina.

PARTICULARS AND PRECAUTIONS

- Creates heat in the body.
- Appropriate any time of day; avoid evening and before bedtime.
- Add block between the thighs as on page 47 to support core and spinal column.
- Add strap around tops of feet or practice one leg at a time to create accessibility.
- Avoid if abdominal or spinal disc issues (anteriorly herniated), acute high blood pressure.
- Full list of Immunity and Whole Health Benefits, page 113.

HOW TO DO IT

Breathe, connect with intention, and visualize pose before doing.

- Start prone on the belly, forehead down, arms by the side, with feet hip-width and parallel to each other.
- Reach the arms behind the back; activate the core to stabilize the upper back and spine.
- Bend the knees, flex the feet, and reach back to hold onto the outer ankles or the feet.
- Hug the thighs into hip-width apart; if you splay them, draw them back to alignment.
- If there is any pain, stop and return to straight legs and clasped hands of Locust Pose C-Clasp.
- Stabilize and deepen Ujjayi breath.
- Create length in the low back by drawing buttocks toward the knees while hugging thighs to hip-width.
- Firm the low belly while still lifting to gently open the body, lengthening all four sides of torso and neck.
- Breathe for up to five breath cycles; do not over-hold.
- Release body and turn the head to one side.
- Either repeat pose or proceed to transition, supine on to the back with knees bent, feet on floor.

SETU BANDHA
(SET-OO BUN-DAH)
BRIDGE POSE

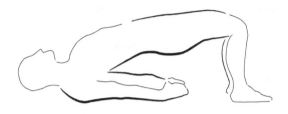

REFRESHING, CLEARING, GENTLY ENERGIZING, CULTIVATES
BREATH EXPANSION

A gateway pose that opens the chest and creates much needed mobility for many of us in the upper back. Opening the chest like opening the window shutters to a fresh air. Inhale and let the breath expand. Exhale and send out the stale air, the held tensions, to release mental, emotional, and physical stress. Vibration and primal sound is a wonderful tool within this posture. Inhale open, exhale OM, AH, UH. It uncaps the pressure and resets the entire system.

STRETCHES (CREATING SPACE)

- Stretches legs, abdomen, spine, chest, lungs, heart, shoulders, entire front body.
- Creates space in abdomen, aiding digestion/elimination and breathing.

STRENGTHENS (CREATING STEADINESS)

- Strengthens legs, buttocks, spine, core, back, shoulders, entire back body.
- Builds energy, courage, and stamina.

PARTICULARS AND PRECAUTIONS

- Creates a gentle heat in the body.
- Appropriate anytime daytime; avoid before bedtime.
- Aids in digestion/elimination and lung capacity.
- Add block between the thighs as on page 47 to support core and spinal column.
- Avoid turning the head; keep neck and head in neutral.
- Avoid if abdominal or spinal disc issues (anteriorly herniated), acute high blood pressure.
- Full list of Immunity and Whole Health Benefits, page 113.

HOW TO DO IT

Breathe, connect with intention, and visualize pose before doing.

- Start reclined supine on the back with the knees bent, feet on the floor, with heels aligned under the knees.
- Align the feet and knees hip-width apart and keep them in this alignment throughout posture.
- Lengthen the arms alongside the torso with the palms face down.
- Refine symmetry in the body so both right and left sides are even along the midline.
- Lengthen through the natural curves of the spine and support the neck curve by drawing the upper back gently in and broadening the chest.
- Root through the feet, hands, back of the shoulders, the head to rebound and lift through hips and chest.
- Stabilize and breathe deeply through the nose.
- Breathe for up to five breath cycles; do not over-hold.
- Release back of hips slowly down to the floor and rest.
- Either repeat pose or proceed to transition to bring Knees into Chest Pose.

APANASANA
(AH-PAH-NAH-SA-NA)
KNEES TO CHEST DETOX PRESS

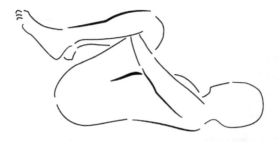

RELEASING, CALMING, DETOXIFYING, AIDS IN ELIMINATION

STRETCHES (CREATING SPACE)

- Stretches the outer hips, buttocks, lower back, shoulders, neck.
- Massages internal organs and abdomen.

STRENGTHENS (CREATING STEADINESS)

- Relaxation and reset of whole body.
- Supports a feeling of stability and calmness.

PARTICULARS AND PRECAUTIONS

- Cools and calms the entire system.
- Aids in digestion and elimination.
- Appropriate any time of day/evening.
- Can be used between other poses as a reset for the system.
- Avoid if pregnant or with abdominal issues.
- Full list of Immunity and Whole Health Benefits, page 113.

Breathe, connect with intention, and visualize pose before doing.

- Start supine on to the back with the feet on the floor, knees best, firm the low belly and lift the heels of the feet until high on the toe tips. This helps stabilize the low back.
- Once stable, exhale, bringing the knees and thighs up into the belly and keeping both head and shoulders anchored to the floor.
- Wrap arms behind the knees, holding onto the forearms or wrists, creating a gentle belly pressure.
- Breathe slowly and fully to massage the internal organs.
- Create a sustainable pressure that is both snug and comfortable.
- Gently rock side to side; explore circular intuitive or freestyle movement.
- If low back and neck feel stable, explore the *parsva*/side version, rolling side to side on slow breaths. Moving side-center-side, massage all areas of the abdomen.
- Massage until it feels right to stop; do not overdo.
- Release knees and feet down to the floor and rest.
- Either repeat pose or proceed to transition into Passive Supine Twist.

JATHARA PARIVARTANASANA
(JAH-TAR-AH PAR-E-VAR-TAH-NAH-SA-NA)
PASSIVE SUPINE TWIST

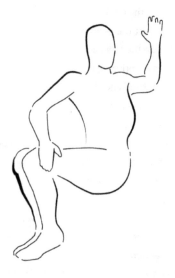

COOLING, CLEARING, QUIETING, AIDS IN ELIMINATION

Twists aid in digestive health, elimination, and spinal health and creates focus. In this passive surrender twist, focus on being gently cleared and wrung out. Allow the body to be breathed by the atmospheric pressure of the earth and life.

STRETCHES (CREATING SPACE)

- Stretches outer hips, side waist, spine, chest, shoulders.
- Massages internal organs and abdomen.

STRENGTHENS (CREATING STEADINESS)

- Creates feeling of calm, can be soothing and quieting.

- Cooling to the body and mind.
- Aids in digestion and elimination.
- Can be practiced anytime.
- Avoid if abdominal or spinal disc issues.
- Full list of Immunity and Whole Health Benefits, page 113.

HOW TO DO IT

Breathe, connect with intention, and visualize pose before doing.

- Start supine, on the back with the feet on the floor, knees bent; firm the low belly and lift the heels of the feet until high on the toe tips. This helps stabilize the low back.
- Once stable, exhale, bringing the knees and thighs up into the belly and keeping both head and shoulders anchored to the floor.
- Breathe slowly and fully to massage the internal organs.
- Keeping the knees bent, exhale, lowering the leg structure to the left side of the body on the floor.
- Inhale, opening the chest toward the sky and drawing the right shoulder down to the floor.
- Release the effort of the twist here; breathe slowly, fluidly, while drawing the top hip down away from the shoulders and twisting the spine.
- Engage the belly muscles and hug thighs together just enough to feel stabilizing and satisfying.
- If sustainable for the neck, turn the head away from the legs.
- Breathe deeply five-plus cycles of breath.
- Firm the low belly, return to center, stabilize, and then proceed to do the other side; equal time/quality.
- Come back to feet on the floor, breathe deeply, and feel the effects of the postures.

CHAPTER 7

PRANAYAMA AND MEDITATION FOR DETOXIFICATION

The breathing exercises in this chapter relax the body, clear mental-emotional tension, and support the lungs in clearing out stale air to bring fresh oxygen in more effectively. A theme with many of the breathing practices in this chapter is the focus on exhalation. When we stretch the exhalation, we force deeply accumulated stagnant air out of the lungs, making room for increased oxygen levels as well as toning the diaphragm and lungs.

In a layered healing approach, we started with the postural detoxification and then move to the more subtle *pranayamas* here. Conscious exhalations support the rest/digest response and, when practiced with awareness and gentle pressure on the belly, stimulate clearing the back of the lungs. If not regularly stimulated, this posterior area of the lungs can become stagnant and be an early place of infection when the immune system is challenged. We want to bring breath, energy, and conscious clearing to the back of the lungs.

EXTEND THE EXHALATION TO LET THE STRESS GO

The use of the exhalation in conjunction with sound vibration can also be very helpful in stress reduction and releasing held emotions such as fear and anger. We are a whole complex being of conscious awareness, the wisdom mind, the organizational mind, our emotions, and physical experience. Our overall resilience and well-being are dependent on an interconnectedness of these layers aligning what we think, how we breathe, and what we do daily. We practice intentional alignment of these layers to fortify our mental/emotional resonance as well as the

RAS—the reticular activating system—response, helping to entrain each breath and exercise to create what you want and clear what you don't want.

NATURAL RELEASES; DON'T SUPPRESS THEM

When these mental-emotional tensions leave the body, there may be a natural release that happens, possibly including tears, laughter, salivation, sweating, belches, hiccups, flatulence, coughing, sneezing, and the like. Do not repress these natural releases. It may be ingrained in you that these releases are to be held in, as it may be considered uncivilized. The impulse to cover or contain these releases may run deep in your habit patterns. I urge you to allow a more primal aspect and simply witness the releases as they come forward. Follow the connections to the root of the release in your physical, mental, and emotional terrain. Then keep deep breathing and move on. Although we do not go deeply into the chakra system of the subtle body in this book, it is foundational to the whole-being health approach shared here and, at the end of this book, there are resources on how to follow these breadcrumbs of whole-being alignment and releases. Look under the Mental-Emotional Yogic Support section and Chakras in the reference section.

These wholistic breathing practices are excellent for boosting cognitive function as well as lung health and are often recommended for those who suffer from asthma or chronic obstructive pulmonary disease as a form of pulmonary rehabilitation. Throughout my twenties, I suffered from chronic anxiety and asthma, and each would feed the other's intensity. Over years of consistent practice of the exercises I share here, along with additional diet and lifestyle changes, I am thankful to report that I no longer experience regular wheezing or shortness of breath, and my default state is now one of steadiness and joy. The magic is in the consistent daily practice, letting go of the outcome, and the patience to witness the shifts. I hope these breathing tools support you as they have me.

IMMUNITY AND WHOLE HEALTH BENEFITS OF FOLLOWING EXERCISES

- Contraction of diaphragm, creating deep detoxification effects.
- Increases oxygen intake and decrease carbon dioxide/debris/stale air.
- Increases blood oxygen and lymphatic and digestive circulation.
- Increases lung/diaphragm strength and elasticity.
- Decreases stress overdrive functions, heart rate, blood pressure, and inflammation.
- Stimulates the vagus nerve, activating the rest/digest response (description on page 66)
- Mindful repetitions support slowing of brain waves and calming the mind.
- Cultivates present-moment awareness, supporting focus, concentration, mental/emotional balance.
- Supports self-regulation, resilience, endurance, and whole-system balance.
- Reduces anxiety, depression, fatigue, brain fog, and feelings of overwhelm.
- With intention, focuses the RAS on positive healing outcome.
- Activates vital energy currents in the body, increasing health, vitality, and radiance.

PRACTICES FOR DETOXIFICATION

VISAMA VRITTI
(VEE-SAH-MA VREE-TEE)
IMBALANCED BREATH EXHALE FOCUS

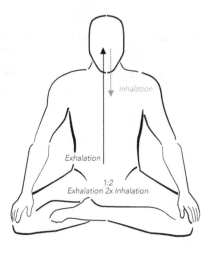

Inhalation

Exhalation

1:2
Exhalation 2x Inhalation

CLEARING, CALMING, STRENGTHENS BREATHING ORGANS

This 1:2 breathing technique can be applied anywhere in your life where you could use to let go, slow down, and allow your system to balance. I personally found this breathing practice helpful in my journey as a mother of three children. I was thankful to have healthy pregnancies, and yet a recurring issue was having high blood pressure readings at the beginning of my regular prenatal checkups. It became something that I dreaded and would experience anxiety over. I began to practice this imbalanced exhale-focused breathing in the waiting room of the doctor's office, and on those days, my blood pressure was significantly lower when tested. I found that even just a handful of rounds as the cuff was on my arm would create a positive effect from one consecutive check to another. It continued to be a game-changer throughout my mothering, as it was helpful during labor in relaxing my mind and body, and essential during early breastfeeding and well beyond into supporting a sometimes-hectic home life. This one is great to have in your back pocket and definitely teach it to your loved ones.

PARTICULARS AND PRECAUTIONS

- Cultivates focus, balance, and relaxation.
- Appropriate any time of day/evening.
- Can be incorporated with Ujjayi breaths.
- Good for restoratives where spine is supported, no core engagement needed; avoid in vigorous poses.
- Cultivate the 1:2 ratio length without undo effort or strain.
- Full list of Immunity and Whole Health Benefits, page 113.

HOW TO DO IT

Stabilize body, elongate spine, cultivating balance; sitting or reclined position can be used.

- Begin to direct the breath out the nostrils and, upon inhaling, feel the coolness of the air move into the nasal openings.
- Exhale the breath completely out and slowly begin to take in the inhalation through the nose while calmly noting the length of the breath.
- Create a sustainable fullness in the inhalation, and then begin to slowly send the exhalation out the nostrils for twice the length of the inhalation.
- Start simply with the ratio of 3-count inhalation to a 6-count exhalation, then build to 4:8, eventually 5:10. Never strain to extend the breath.
- At the end of the exhalation, firm the lowest part of the low belly and gently push the remaining air out.
- Cultivate a balance of effort and passivity and avoid any strain or over-ambition.

CHANDRA BHEDANA
(CHAHN-DRAH BED-AH-NA)
LEFT NOSTRIL DOMINANCE BREATH

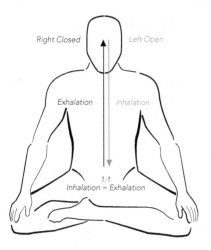

CALMING, STABILIZING, CULTIVATES RECEPTIVITY AND CREATIVITY

Almost like a magic button of calming, closing off the right nostril to create dominance in the left is like drinking a cool glass of water on a hot day. It calms, cools, and creates a relaxation reset. I have found this especially helpful when I am revved up with to-dos and in an edgy, agitated state. For me, it doesn't take long to feel a shift, and, as with many of these foundational breathing techniques, it can be done anywhere and anytime (as long as you are not driving or operating heavy machinery).

PARTICULARS AND PRECAUTIONS

- Stabilizes, calms, and reduces tension.
- Left nostril stimulation increases right brain (receptivity/creativity) brain activity.
- Appropriate any time of day/evening.

- Cultivate the 1:1 or 1:2 ratio length without undue effort or strain.
- Full list of Immunity and Whole Health Benefits, page 113.

Full list of Immunity and Whole Health Benefits, page 113.

HOW TO DO IT

Stabilize body, elongate spine, cultivating balance; sitting or reclined position can be used.

- Begin to direct the breath out the nostrils and upon inhaling feel the coolness of the air move into the nasal openings.
- Exhale the breath completely out and slowly begin to take in the inhalation through the nose while calmly noting the length of the breath.
- Create a sustainable fullness in the inhalation and then begin to slowly send the exhalation out the nostrils for the same length and with the same vigor.
- With the dominant-hand middle finger, gently press close the right nostril at the end of the cartilage, just before the crease of the nasal flare.
- With steady, consistent pressure, keep that nostril closed during the entirety of the rounds of practice.
- Exhale and inhale through the left nostril completely and begin to create a Sama Vritti and Full Complete breath, isolating the left nostril only.
- Do three rounds of six to eight repetitions of this Chandra Bhedana, or as many as feels clearing and calming.
- Sit in quiet stillness, breathing evenly and naturally through both nostrils, before transitioning.

KAPALABHATI
(KAH-PAH-LAH-BAH-TEE)
SHINING SKULL KRIYA (MEDIUM TEMPO)

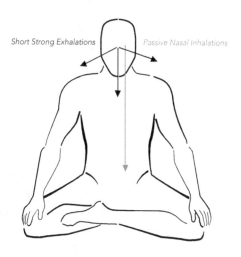

Short Strong Exhalations   *Passive Nasal Inhalations*

CLEARING, BALANCING, MIMICS SNEEZING FOR DETOXIFICATION

Here we are mimicking sneezing (when utilizing the nose) and coughing (when utilizing the mouth) with our breaths, and there is a direct stimulation of the abdominals, lungs, throat, and sinus cavities. There are a multitude of variations of this practice and each amplifies a different aspect of detoxification. Shining Skull Breath is shared in the seminal yogic text the *Hatha Yoga Pradipika*, as one of the six essential cleansing techniques or Shat Kriyas, which is why I categorized it as a kriya versus a pranayama. Regardless of how you categorize it, it is an essential practice, and one that can be adapted to many needs.

In this variation, we will practice at a medium tempo with the exhalations clearing through the nasal passages, mimicking a sneeze. When exhalations are drawn out long and slow, it calms the system as well as clearing it. The faster the repetitions of breaths, the more energizing and warming it becomes. Consider time of day and personal state of being, as well as current season, to prescribe the ideal tempo for you here. Note more support on how to choose the best tempo for *Kapalabhati Kriya* below on page 47.

PARTICULARS AND PRECAUTIONS

- Pushes out stale air and debris from deep in the lungs.
- Contracts deep areas of diaphragm, supporting detox in lower abdominal cavity.
- Appropriate for morning to late afternoon, depending on the tempo of exhalations.
- Cultivate the ratio length to a length that feels steady yet spacious without undue effort; never strain.
- Avoid in evening and before bedtime.
- Avoid pushing for volume on vocal cords, and only practice as feels sustainable.
- Avoid breath practice if experiencing instability or lightheadedness.
- Avoid with high blood pressure, heart issues, epilepsy, hernia, recent abdominal surgery, or if pregnant.
- Full list of Immunity and Whole Health Benefits, page 113.

HOW TO DO IT

Stabilize body, elongate spine, cultivating balance; sitting position is recommended.

- Become aware of the breath and create balanced repetitions.
- Begin a slow, forceful exhalation through the nose with the mouth closed, while creating a slight constriction in the throat similar to Ujjayi Breath, page 82.
- Allow the inhalation to drop in automatically while focusing effort on strong and consistent exhalations, originating from deep in the lower abdomen, forcing air past the throat, sinuses and out of the nose.
- Cultivate the extended the exhalation out a three-to-five-count stretch, which is a medium tempo and will create a balanced mind and energy quality.

- Repeat for about a thirty-second increment for three rounds or as long as it feels sustainable.
- Once completed, sit quietly, breathing, allowing for a natural cadence and quality of breath.
- Notice if the breath automatically slows and settles into an effortless pause and natural retention.
- Enjoy these effortless retentions as they are a gateway into a deep quiet and relaxation.

TEMPOS OF KAPALABHATI KRIYA

five-to-seven-count extended exhalation (slow)	Creates a calming, cooling clearing effect.
three-to-five-count length exhalation (medium)	Creates a balancing clearing effect.
one-to-two-count exhalation (fast)	Creates an energizing, heating clearing effect.

SIMHASANA KRIYA
(SIM-HAH-SAH-NA KREE-YA)
LION'S CLEANSING MUDRA

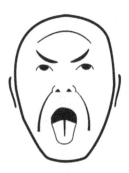

CLEARING, STRESS-RELIEVING, CULTIVATES COURAGE

In the classic Hatha Yoga text *Gheranda Samhita*, Simhasana or Lion's Breath is described as the "destroyer of disease." The practice that unblocks the passage of rejuvenation and flow of life. In the *Hatha Yoga Pradipika*, this breath is mentioned as one of the four most excellent of all yoga postures for beneficial effects on the whole being. For me it has been invaluable in clearing out tensions of daily life. I have found it is practically adaptable and can be practiced kneeling, as well as in cross-legged seat as it is often instructed, as well as in other, more active clearing asanas such as Utkatasana/Thunderbolt or other detox postures in this chapter. The lion represents the power of raw emotion and the roaring as clearing that emotion to make way for higher processing, peace, and healing. Here we deeply expand the lungs and stretch the throat and tongue to activate from the perineum to the midbrain, as this lion's roar clears the multilayered tensions that we accumulate in the body.

PARTICULARS AND PRECAUTIONS

- Firms and tones the platysma muscle in the neck and face.
- Stimulates the abdominal cavity, throat, thyroid gland, vocal cords, tongue, and sinuses.
- Pushes out stale air particles from the deeper areas of the lungs, throat, and mouth.
- Appropriate for morning to late afternoon; avoid before bedtime.
- Avoid pushing for volume on vocal cords, and only practice as feels sustainable.
- Avoid breath practice if experiencing instability or lightheadedness.
- Avoid if neck or throat injury, high blood pressure, heart issues, epilepsy, hernia, or recent abdominal surgery.
- Full list of Immunity and Whole Health Benefits, page 113.

HOW TO DO IT

Stabilize body, elongate spine, cultivating balance; sitting position is recommended.

- Become aware of the breath and create balanced repetitions.
- Stretch the tongue out of the mouth, down toward the chin as far as it will go, while making a HAH sound, drawing the belly up and in to empty the lungs completely.
- Focus the eyes up in between the eyebrows. It is okay if the eye focus creates a crossing of the eyes.
- Inhale through the nose and relax the eye gaze as you take in breath.
- Repeat three to six times until you feel a cleared, calm, alert state. Avoid excessive pressure on the vocal cords.
- Focus on the upward lift of the low belly and full release of the breath out of the lungs.
- Sit quietly, breathing evenly through the nostrils, observe how you feel, and create balance.

TONGUE POSITIONS FOR SIMHASANA KRIYA/LION'S BREATH

Another variation of Lion's Breath that I utilize when I am needing a quick reset that feels immediately calming to the nervous system is using the tongue tip at the back of the bottom teeth, creating leverage to pull the root of the tongue more strongly out of the throat. The root of the tongue connects directly into the vagus nerve, directly into the rest/digest response, and can be a direct gateway to relaxing the whole body when released. This variation puts less stretch on the neck and more stretch on the back of the tongue, which directly connects to the lymph and the lingual tonsils, creating extra stimulation there and arguably boosting our immune defense as well. Consider trying both variations and experiencing the effects.

THE *DRISHTI* (DRISH-TEE) OR EYE FOCUS AREAS OF LION'S BREATH.

1. Third Eye or between the eyebrows. This focus brings energy and awareness to the frontal lobe and is considered to open inner vision and expanded intuitive insight.
2. Tip of the nose, entrance of the nasal flares, and nostrils, to activate the polar energies *ida* and *pingala nadi*, which open and balance the central channels of energy supporting the rise of creative life force through the system.

BAKURA KRIYA
(BAH-KOO-RAH KREE-YA)
TRUMPET OR PURSED LIP CLEANSING

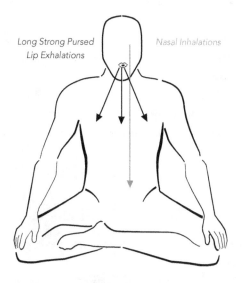

Long Strong Pursed Lip Exhalations

Nasal Inhalations

CLEARING, STRESS-RELIEVING, DETOXIFIES LUNGS

You may or may not find this particular kriya in an ancient yogic text, yet it is potent and a game-changer. The strong, sustained-exhalation breathing is a great way to strengthen the diaphragm and the lungs as well as clear the lungs of stagnant air and toxins. If making trumpet sounds is not your thing, exhale out as if slowly blowing out a set of birthday candles and get similar benefits. The American Lung Association utilizes a version of this they refer to as Pursed Lip Breathing as a pulmonary rehabilitation tool. As a Miles Davis fan, I have often played my air trumpet (to my children's embarrassment) and discovered I could incorporate my super fun pretend trumpet with some deep cleansing of my lungs. The lung benefits are many, and my children's reaction gave me a hearty laugh, which inspired me to play my "trumpet" for them even more. Ultimately, laughing is one of our greatest medicines, and if this potent clearing breath leads you to laughter, consider it the highest level of immune support available.

PARTICULARS AND PRECAUTIONS

- Stimulates the abdominal cavity, throat, thyroid gland, vocal cords, tongue, and sinuses.
- Pushes out stale air particles from the deeper areas of the lungs, throat, and mouth.
- Appropriate for morning to late afternoon; avoid before bedtime.
- Avoid pushing for volume on vocal cords and only practice as feels sustainable.
- Avoid breath practice if experiencing instability or lightheadedness.
- Avoid if neck or throat injury, history of high blood pressure, heart problems, epilepsy, hernia, or recent abdominal surgery, or if pregnant.
- Full list of Immunity and Whole Health Benefits, page 113.

HOW TO DO IT

Stabilize body, elongate spine, cultivating balance; sitting position is recommended.

- Become aware of the breath and create balanced repetitions.
- Inhale through the nostrils, preparing for an energized exhalation, slowly and completely through the pursed lips, creating a humming trumpet-like sound. Or simply exhale as if blowing out a set of birthday candles.
- Continuing breathing through the nose and creating pursed exhales out the mouth with no tonality or in a tune that feels delightful to you.
- The key is to extend the exhalations out as far as you can without strain.
- Firm the low belly in and up at the very end of the exhalation to get the last bit of air to come out.
- Utilize your inner vision to see all the toxins being sent out by each extended exhalation.
- Repeat for a minimum of one minute, a maximum of five minutes; consider repeating for three rounds.
- Afterward, sit quietly, breathing evenly through the nostrils; observe how you feel and create balance.

A flute, a balloon, a straw, or repeatedly counting to ten to the end of an exhale are other ways to create similar benefits of this exercise. You can actually play a wind instrument (I pretend to play a trumpet and play a real flute to create the same benefits), or repetitively blow up a balloon or blow through a straw for five to ten minutes each day. Or, work as described in the highly recommended book by James Nestor, *Breath*, where he suggests utilizing a repetitive counting of ten until there is no more exhale to utilize. Whatever tool you utilize, it works wonders in strengthening and detoxing the lungs and pulmonary system.

KIRTAN KRIYA
(KEER-TAN KREE-YA)
SINGING MEDITATION

SA TA NA MA KRIYA

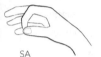
SA

TA

NA

MA

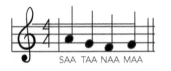
SAA TAA NAA MAA

CLEARING, CALMING, ENHANCES COGNITIVE FUNCTION

Kirtan translates as singing, *kriya* as cleansing technique, and this clearing meditation is my go-to when I am anxious and having difficulty staying still. I have found multiple variations of this *kriya* to be effective and the full practice, running thirty minutes, to be intense in endurance as well as delivering dramatic mental, emotional, and energetic effects.

I first learned this practice through studying the teachings of Yogi Bhajan in the kundalini yoga tradition, and over the years I have passed it on in a shortened version to both children and adults. To my inspiration, I have received feedback from many friends using this practice to guide them peacefully through great challenges such as rounds of chemotherapy or lengthy MRI (no movement usage here) to successfully abate claustrophobia. It can be adapted for many helpful purposes.

The key helpful aspects of this practice are the extended repetitions to focus and quiet the mind, visualization between the eyebrows that stimulates the frontal lobe, and the marrying of simple mudras (hand gestures) with mantras (the sounds of Sa Ta Na Ma, which derive from Sat Nam or "I am" or "The truth of my essence") that stimulate key areas of the brain and upper soft palate at the roof of the mouth.

As shared in the *Journal of Alzheimer's Disease*,[2] twelve minutes of Kirtan Kriya practiced daily improves memory, cognitive function and mitigates neurodegeneration in the prevention of Alzheimer's disease. They found that Kirtan Kriya reduced inflammation, anxiety, and depression, and improved memory, sleep, and the immune system.

Along with these physical and mental benefits, Kirtan Kriya also activates multiple energy healing points and channels throughout the body. We activate these key *marma*, or acupressure points, with the tongue as well as with the tips of the fingers as we move through the mudras or energy seals in repetition. This truly is a whole-being healing power practice!

On SA, press index finger pad to thumb pad on each hand.
On TA, press middle finger pad to thumb pad on each hand.
On NA, press ring finger pad to thumb pad on each hand.
On MA, press pinky finger pad to thumb pad on each hand.

PARTICULARS AND PRECAUTIONS

- Supports cognitive function, memory, and good-quality sleep.
- Stimulates the abdominal cavity, throat, thyroid gland, vocal cords, tongue, and sinuses.
- Pushes stale air particles out of the deeper areas of the lungs, throat, and mouth.
- Appropriate for morning to late afternoon; avoid before bedtime.
- Avoid pushing for volume on vocal cords and only practice as feels sustainable.
- Full list of Immunity and Whole Health Benefits, page 113.

---

2   https://www.j-alz.com/vol48-1

Stabilize body, elongate spine, cultivating balance; sitting position is recommended.

- Become aware of the breath and create balanced repetitions.
- Bring awareness to the top of the head and the mental image of healing golden light moving down into the crown of the head and gently exiting through the eyebrow center or third eye.
- Hold and reconnect with this image of light and sound movement throughout meditation.
- Inhale through the nostrils as you sing.
- SA TA NA MA in the tones indicated above (or in tonal sequence) in conjunction with the hand mudras.

> *On SA, press index finger pad to thumb pad on each hand.*
> *On TA, press middle finger pad to thumb pad on each hand.*
> *On NA, press ring finger pad to thumb pad on each hand.*
> *On MA, press pinky finger pad to thumb pad on each hand.*

- Repeat out loud in full (yet gentle) voice with mudras for two minutes.
- Repeat out loud in whisper (again gentle, no strain in vocal cords) voice with mudras for two minutes.
- Repeat silently inside, continuing with mudras for four minutes.
- In reverse, repeat in whisper (again gentle, no strain in vocal cords) voice with mudras for two minutes.
- Repeat in full (yet gentle) voice with mudras for two minutes, for a total of twelve minutes.
- Sit quietly, breathing naturally, observing how you feel, and resetting in the fullness.

TIMINGS OF SEGMENTS OF KIRTAN KRIYA

Timings taught by Yogi Bhajan (thirty-one-minute duration)
- Five-minute Full Voice
- Five-minute Whisper Voice
- Ten-minute Vibration of Silent Repetition
- Five-minute Whisper
- Five-minute Full voice
- One-minute Silent Stillness

Cognitive Benefit Recommended (twelve-minute duration)
- Two-minute Full Voice
- Two-minute Whisper Voice
- Four-minute Vibration in Silent Repetition
- Two-minute Whisper Voice
- Two-minute Full Voice
- One-minute Silent Stillness

Mini Reset Version (seven-minute duration)
- One-minute Full Voice
- One-minute Whisper Voice
- Two-minute Vibration in Silent Repetition
- One-minute Whisper Voice
- One-minute Full Voice
- One-minute Silent Stillness

CHAPTER 8

SEQUENCES FOR DETOXIFICATION

Step by step, we continue to build, adding on in understanding, intention, new tools, and refining previous ones. This chapter, similar to Chapter 4 in Part I, weaves together key practices for simple daily actionable sequences.

Again, the intention is to get you moving and doing. I hope that you collaborate with me and use these as a jumping-off point, then feel your way intuitively into additional body movements that deepen your experience.

The sequences that follow are a sampling of what is possible to support you to continue to build a daily practice.

The following sequences are in this order

1. Three-Minute Daily Essential Detox Sequence
2. Eight-Minute Daily Essential +Detox Combination Sequence
3. Detoxification Practice Sequence
4. Detoxification Breathing Sequence

#1
THREE-MINUTE DAILY ESSENTIAL DETOX SEQUENCE

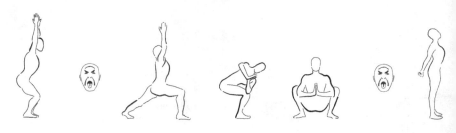

#2
EIGHT-MINUTE DAILY ESSENTIAL + DETOX COMBINATION SEQUENCE

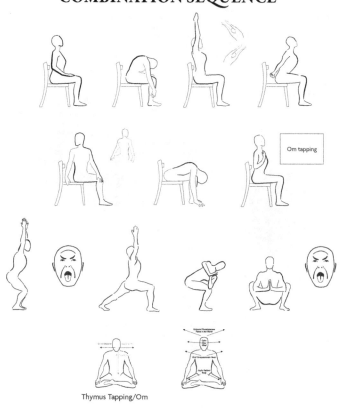

Om tapping

Thymus Tapping/Om

#3
DETOXIFICATION PRACTICE SEQUENCE

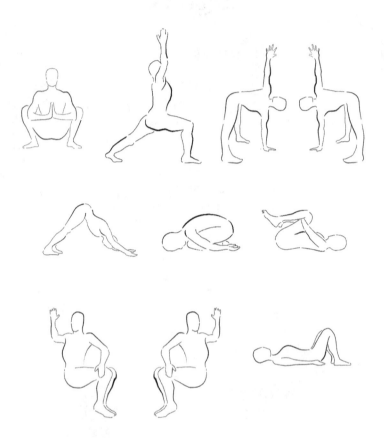

#4
DETOXIFICATION BREATHING SEQUENCE

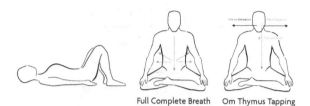

Full Complete Breath   Om Thymus Tapping

Visama Vritti Exhale Focus   Prone Full Complete Breaths

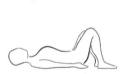

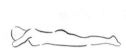

Reclined Expansive 3 Part Inhalation

Chandra Bhedana:
Left Nostril Dominance

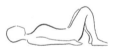

SA TA NA MA KRIYA

SA   TA   NA   MA

SAA TAA NAA MAA

"ONLY ONE THING? DO THIS."

Chapter 5

Address one area of stress in your life. Make one micro change and repeat it consistently.

Chapter 6

Rotate the spine and compress abdominal cavity each day to aid detoxing the body.

Do

Knees to Chest   Supine Spinal Twist Daily

Chapter 7

Kirtan Kriya/Singing Meditation, page 154.

SA TA NA MA KRIYA

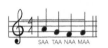

SA   TA   NA   MA   SAA TAA NAA MAA

Chapter 8

Three-Minute Daily Essential Detox Sequence

PART III

INTEGRATION

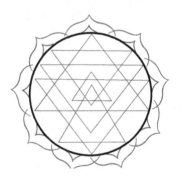

CHAPTER 9

FOCUS AND FREEDOM FOR INTEGRATION

It is the *how* we do what we do that makes a difference. It is the intention and direction of the focus that will boost healing or the opposite, reduce the potency.

What we focus on and how we direct our attention is the transforming aspect of this practice. It moves it from simple calisthenics or breathing to whole-life positive transformation. If you practice with a sense of pressure, ambition, or desperation, you will not create the same experience or outcome as if you practice with a relaxed dedication and consistency, with trust in the process.

Whatever you put your focus on will expand. That place of attention will grow and become stronger. With the clarity and stability you have created here, you will have an easier time redirecting yourself to place your attention on only what you want to continue—guiding yourself to what you want, instead of what you don't want or are worried about.

Now, I can imagine, if you are an earnest student, that at this point there may be the potential for overwhelm. Therefore, I am here wholeheartedly to guide you to trust the explorations and to let the pull to *feel good* guide you.

There is a momentum of life-giving energy when we consistently redirect our focus to a sense of ease and joy. There is a palpable healing with the emotion of joy, and wherever you can conjure that into your day and practice, you will turbo-boost the effects. To be clear, I am not saying to not do the things that are hard. I am saying, do what needs to be done, and do it with your heart mind on possibility and positive outcome. Fear and resistance will drain you. The possibility mindset and joy will boost you.

This extra boost within the power of positive emotions is a release of a group of happy hormones, dopamine, serotonin, oxytocin, and endorphins. We have been purposely cultivating this quartet of happy hormones with all of our movements, breaths, meditations, and intention focus. We have been working toward creating a positive feedback loop that will help you *want* to return to do the things that will help you thrive. We have been relying on that innate tendency to want to go toward what is easy and pleasurable and away from what is difficult and painful.

Focus on feeling good and what feels accessible to practice. Repeat those practices until they become so integrated in you that it feels almost effortless. Ride on the positive feedback loop and allow the success momentum to affirm you forward. As we know, struggle begets struggle, so practice simply catching the struggle and breathing it out. Take the struggle out of your poses, your breathing, your meditation, your cooking, your parenting, your self-care—out of all of it.

This practice of redirecting and shifting personal mindset from negative to positive is one of the most difficult personal practices that I have found. Because of the level of challenge, I refer to it as fierce kindness. It takes an intensity of clarity, commitment, and truthfulness, coupled with compassion and unconditional love, to master this practice. The mastery comes from consistency and nonattachment or taking the struggle out.

We know that there is power in repetition and consistency, which is why we have been spending the time bringing awareness to our habits. This consistency coupled with ease or nonattachment is called *abhyasa* (AH-bee-YAH-sah) and *vairagya* (VAY-RAH-gyah), and it is a key to whole health integration.

I call it *Keep going/Oh well,* and I use it as a mantra to help instantaneously reset and move myself forward without struggle.

Cultivate that freedom within yourself by utilizing the potent practice of "keep going" and "oh well." You stumbled? Oh well! Brush yourself off and keep going. You missed a day? Oh well, don't beat yourself up, simply start again the next day. They are a beautiful couple that are not to be separated. Too much *keep going* creates rigidity, too much *oh well* and there is a lack of vitality. Our job is to dance within the balance.

The body, mind, emotions, and our vitality are constantly changing. Each day and time of life will call for a different incarnation of this practice to help bring these aspects of self to harmony. It is harmony that will boost our immune function and whole health. Only through trial and error, trial and delightful success, will this delicate harmony be created.

There may be the occasion when your mind clearly understands the information being shared, yet your body has not experienced the feeling or effect, and you hesitate to practice. There may be an occasion when your body remembers the feel-good experience of the movements and breath, yet emotionally you feel too sad or angry to get on the mat. This is the time we return to self-study. What is this pain or resistance trying to tell me? This is where we slow down and tune into the subtle clues and go back to our tools of listening to see what is being revealed. As this practice is circular, not linear, we begin again and continue to inquire "What is this here to teach me?" and "How can I learn from this and utilize this clarity for nourishment?"

When you are suffering, ask yourself, "What am I denying right now?" Once you have given the suppressed sensation, emotion, or awareness its time to be heard, it will begin to shift. Acknowledge the need or unmet desire underneath the feeling. Then return your attention to your *intention* and the focus of creation and feeling good. Only once we have acknowledged the pain, the feelings of separation, realized that the other is not the other, but us. That we live within in all things and all things live within us. It is only then that we can move on its shoulders to transmuting that energy into healing.

The more you practice this process of pausing to feel, listen, and then choose to do based on a possibility and solution mindset, the easier it becomes. The more automatic and integrated into your personality and habits the greater the outcome. Affirm and learn, as your brain's neuroplasticity is ageless, and it has the ability to rewrite itself. You have the power to create new helpful habits, as the sheer repetition of thinking a thought, creating a feeling, and doing an action will rewire the brain and transform your life.

As you do your yoga and address the root causes of stress and dis-ease, you will rehab your nervous system and amplify your longevity functions.

Within the previous chapters, we have built a stable scaffold of understanding. The rest of this book is to support you in doing your practice, getting you over the possible hurdles to practicing, and inspiring you to get curious and begin to add new tools into your yogic toolbox. Consider these chapters in Part III as a playground of exploration for vitality and an entry into a more intricate practice. The healing magic of yoga can only be unlocked when it is *practiced*. Revel in the aspect, that this is a practice, not a performance. Practice is purposely imperfect, and the imperfect nature of your practice is just right and perfect.

As we focus on integrating the actual doing of our practice, I've included here some helpful strategies that I have learned and utilize in my own life. A few of them we have visited previously in other chapters, yet I include them here to support their importance and fortify you integrating them. I am consistently revising and upgrading my systems of how I do things and I hope that, as you explore these, they inspire you to do the same.

STRATEGIES TO HELP YOU DO YOUR HEALING PRACTICES

Prepare, make a plan, write it, speak it (*Awareness-Intention-Action-Manifestation*) Think about what you will do, write it down, create the support, and then repeat it with success. An example could be:

The need is this...
My intention is this...
I will do this...
It will feel like this...

First-minute follow-through with mental rehearsal. As you get fluent in utilizing your imagination and mental rehearsal in this way, it will become fast and efficient. See yourself step by step leading up to and doing your practice in your mind's eye. It is not necessary to mentally rehearse the entire practice to be effective, I have found the first minute to be helpful for follow-through. This is how I start my day (every day), while still in bed, I do mindful breathing, connect with my intentions, and then mentally rehearse the key first minute of whatever I am focusing on or that has some challenge for my day.

Double down on the micro practices. By now I know you are clear, it is the little things we do each day that have the greatest accumulative effect. So give that mini practice all your attention. Pick a mini practice and do it every day for healing effect. For example, practice doing a forward fold seated on your chair, and while there, practice five Full Complete Breaths (page 77), and then sit up and do a seated rotation before working on the computer, or practice the Intention-Setting Meditation Affirmations before getting out of the bed each morning and just before you fall asleep each night.

Easy to remember and to accomplish. Create reminders and strategies so your practice is super easy to do. Keep the meditation cushion in view. Set up your props and mat so they are ready to go. Prepare the night before, so it is ready for you the next morning. Put up a big reminder note to *breathe* at eye level. Reset your mat and props for the next time immediately after practicing so you are ready. Put the energy in preparation so it is minimal effort to do successfully every day.

Fun and Feel Good. Support that positive feedback loop that we have been exploring. Consider adding an extra sales boost by narrating out loud the positive habit as you do it. "Now I'm aligning my spine to make room for my internal organs, supporting my lungs' expansion, and boosting my immune system." Say it out loud and with delight, believe it and enjoy the process.

Add it on top of another successful habit. This is what James Clear, the author of *Atomic Habits*, refers to as habit stacking, and it is one of my favorite strategies. Stack the new practice on top of an already ingrained habit, such as using the bathroom, making the bed, walking the dog, or sitting at your desk. What do you do every day, already, like clockwork? Add a mini yoga practice on top of it.

Re-set up the habit as you finish it. This one I find super helpful, and I find that the reset right after I finish is much more efficient than if I start cold the next day. It does naturally incorporate a brief mental rehearsal while the reset is happening, which is a part of its effectiveness.

Get really good at easy and then add a little more. Start with the practices that are totally in your wheelhouse. Enjoy and celebrate the success of those. Then let it inspire you to take another *little* habit more. Before you know it, you will have created an amazing health and life change, just by adding one little easy step at a time. Remember, we are creating healing from joy, not pain, so make the small choices throughout the day that mirror, reflect, and materialize that for yourself.

As my husband teases: more milk, less moo. Although planning and discussion of preparation for your practice may be helpful, the essence of the practice is *skill in action*, and that comes from doing. So less mooing around and more *doing*. Come on, move with me; pause, put the book down, or if you are listening, pause the recording, and stand up. Big breath and do a Sun Stretch, then twist the spine and now forward fold...okay back in, how was that? Felt great over here!

Unless *moo* is actually what is needed. Sometimes, when there is emotional resistance or hesitance, sound clearing, or toning, is exactly what is needed to release the held tension. Is that feeling stuck in your gut, your chest, or your throat? The action of the moo is needed then, or in this case a big sigh or primal AH sound, until you are ready to get doing. There are some excellent toning exercises in Chapter 11 coming up! When you practice these sound-based toning practices, give it your all. Create a safe space where you feel comfortable making a full sound. A sound that opens the channels of clearing and remember that natural clearing can look like crying, laughing, sneezing, coughing, hiccups, flatulence, salivation, and more! Please don't suppress these natural releases, *moooo* them out.

Teach as you learn. Don't wait until you are a master. Start now, as you are learning. I bet there is someone who could greatly benefit from a *Full Complete Breath* or the *Daily Essential Mini Practice*. Teach them and do it with them. They will receive a gift and you will get clearer by teaching them. It will create confidence and positive healing energy moving forward for you both.

As the above are strategies on how to add more practice into your life, the following are some strategies to subtract a habit or tendency that isn't supporting your health.

Complicate it, make it a hassle or hard to do. If it is watching too much TV, for example, lock away the remote in the farthest cabinet so it is a hassle to get to. Whoever may be your accomplice in this habit, declare to them your intention and ask them to support you by not helping you do the tendency.

Declare how it obviously gross it is. Narrate out loud the bad habit as you do it. "Now I am pouring this poisonous glass of wine, that has tons of pesticides in it, destroying my liver and making me feel like shit." Hmmm, appetizing, much harder to do now.

"May the just-the-right-amount-of-force be with you." Replace the negative self-talk with positive to give you an energy boost. Instead of "I have to exercise, and I don't want to," say "I am grateful I can move my body." Instead of "I can't meditate," try "I breathe to relax my mind." Instead of" I'm not flexible," try "I'm making space in my very stable body." try" It feels wonderful to take care of myself and do my practice." When I shift my inner dialogue out of lack, and I move to possibility, I get a surge of energy, or a little force to get me moving through resistance, and to all my fellow Jedi in training, may the *just-the-right-amount-of-force* be with you.

Replace the habit with a new positive one that supports the base need. Similar to switching the negative thought to a positive one. Taking the wine example from above, I look at what that dinnertime glass of wine may be giving me, and let's say that it is a feeling of festivity or breaking up the mundane—then I may still use a wine glass but replace wine with sparkling water with a twist of lime, to create the better-for-me festivity upgrade. In my yoga practice, it could be catching myself when I push my body into struggle, for example holding Plank Pose past sustainability, and choosing to replace that plank with Child's Pose to create pleasure instead of punishment.

Whole-being harmony is not a static destination. It is a daily journey of falling out of harmony and getting back in. Some days there will be little resistance to practicing, and other days it may be much more difficult. That is the dance of energy and of life.

The great news is that like with any habit, the more we do it, the easier it gets. It can become an automatic process that becomes effortless. If we create solid systems for ourselves that have clear effective tools, a rooted understanding of why, when, and how to use them, connected into our truest self, we will have power in our transformation.

Let's keep going.

CHAPTER 10

ASANAS FOR INTEGRATION

Believe in the tipping point.

When you least expect it, there will be a tipping point, when all these small practices will begin a cascade of healing benefits. Stay the course, you will begin to see the accumulative effects of your consistent actions.

With our consistency, we are now cooking with gas as we begin to layer in additional, sometimes more complex, practices with the foundation of what we created. One pleasure habit loop at a time, we step forward into whole-being health and integration.

The sock, *then the shoe*.

If you put on your shoe and then your sock, you get a very different experience than if you put on sock and then shoe. Sequence matters. Trust this process and the steps that we have put in place for success. Remember, it is not about incorporating every pose in this book or in the encyclopedia of yoga, it is about picking the right one for you, and once that is integrated into a regular supportive habit, stacking another onto it and slowly building a helpful ingrained sequence or life habit.

In this final asana chapter, we are to explore three categories of postures that help support focus on what is important, balanced energy of ease and effort, and purpose-driven expression that feels integrated in a harmonious way. Mind, body, breath, and spirit aligned and woven seamlessly together. At least for the moment anyway again, it is a practice not, a performance of perfect.

In this section, there are very accessible poses for most bodies, and there are also some slightly more challenging postures that rely on a progression of understanding and previous strength-building. Specifically, I am referring to *Pursvottansana* or Reverse Tabletop, *Bound Halasana* or Bound Plough, *Virabhadrasana 3* or Warrior 3, and *Adho Mukha Vriksasana* or Handstand Using a Wall; approach these postures with caution and do not force them, or even do them if you are not feeling calm, steady, and ready.

> "What you focus on expands."
> —*Fierce Kindness; Be a Positive Force for Change*

Focus on guiding the positive healing intention into each breath and movement. Trust the process and take time during and after the finish of each posture to enjoy what you have created.

IMMUNITY BENEFITS FOR THE FOLLOWING FOCUS, FREEDOM, AND INTEGRATION POSTURES

- Aids in cognitive function, balancing hemispheres of the brain.
- Increases coordination, endurance, resilience, and focus.
- Increases oxygen/blood circulation; decreases stagnation and toxins.
- Aids in digestion, breathing, cardiovascular, and brain and glandular function.
- Supports expansion of the diaphragm and the lungs.
- Decreases inflammation and aids in lymphatic drainage.
- Supports the rest/digest response of the parasympathetic nervous system.
- Supports mental/emotional outlook, releasing endorphins, serotonin, and dopamine.
- Increases stamina, endurance, and resilience.
- Creates feelings of release, freedom, focus, courage, and resilience.
- Activates vital energy (pranic) lines through the entire body.

POSES FOR FOCUS

DANDAYAMANA BHARMANASANA
(DAWN-DAH-YA-MAH-NA BAR-MAH-NAH-SAH-NA)
TABLETOP ALTERNATE ARM AND LEG

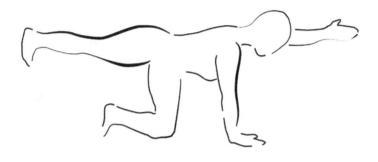

BALANCE, CALMING, CORE AND SPINAL STABILIZER, SUPPORTS
COGNITIVE FUNCTION

A superfood of yoga postures, this tabletop core stabilizer is a powerhouse of balancing for the spine, systems, hemispheres of the brain, and nervous system. This pose is easily adaptable to make it simpler or more complex to be beneficial for every practitioner. Add longer holds and presses within to make it more challenging, or turn it on its back, supine, to take all weight off the limbs. It is a cousin of alternate nostril breathing (page 222) and can be considered as meditation prep, as it supports ease of entry into a meditative state of mind.

STRETCHES (CREATING SPACE)

- Stretches the back of the legs, hips, buttocks, lower back, shoulders, hands, neck.
- Relieves lower back compression when hips stay in neutral position.
- Creates space in abdominal cavity.

- Legs, core, entire spinal column, arms, lungs, heart, and cognitive brain function.
- Increases coordination, stability, and focus.

PARTICULARS AND PRECAUTIONS

- Stabilizes and strengthens spinal column.
- Aids in cognitive function, balancing hemispheres of the brain.
- Appropriate any time of day or evening.
- Add padding under the knees for comfort.
- Avoid if knee or wrist injury; practice supine (on the back) or in a chair.
- Full list of Immunity and Whole Health Benefits, page 173.
- Add dynamic rounding and arching the spine prior to series if there is spinal stiffness.

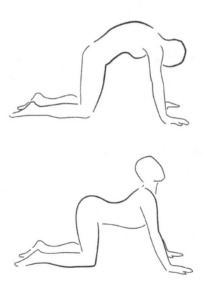

Breathe, connect with intention, and visualize pose before doing.

- Starting on hands/knees, with the shoulders stacked over the wrists and the knees aligned under the hips.
- Align head in line with the shoulders and gaze at one point of focus ahead of the nose.
- Lengthen through side waist so the torso is even on all sides and keeping both hips and shoulders stable.
- Inhale and reach with one arm, palm facing the midline, at shoulder height.
- Engage the core, stabilize torso while reaching the opposite leg directly back, parallel to floor.
- Straighten the leg and press through the heel so leg is parallel to the floor, heel in line with buttocks.
- Square the hips and shoulders and hold to create strength and balance.
- Continue to breathe evenly and stabilize this position for a count of three breaths.
- Simultaneously bring both hand and knee down to the floor at the exact same time.
- Repeat with the other side with the same length of hold.
- Continue to do a minimum of three rounds, up to eight rounds.
- Rest in Child's Pose as seen on page 58.

Create more strength and stability by pressing the heel to the wall. Set up the Tabletop position one leg's distance away from the wall. Press the heel directly back from the hips, parallel to the floor. Avoid lifting the heel higher than the hips, as it can create strain in the lower back, sacral area. Follow the above instructions and activating the buttocks to press the heel into wall.

GARUDASANA
(GAH-ROO-DAH-SAH-NA)
EAGLE POSE

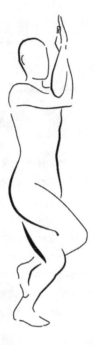

BALANCE, FOCUS, MASSAGES LYMPH NODES, LEG/CORE STRENGTH

What is more important: the cultivation in the nest, or the spreading of the wings to fly? This pose is the practice of drawing in resources and reducing all unnecessary effort to hold balance with grace and stability. Practice to clear out the needless and focus the attention on what is essential to be balanced and healthy, to be able to take flight. Allow the great eagle to give you focus and power to spread your wings and *on the energy of inspiration*, fly. Please note that Eagle and Soaring Eagle go together on one side, and then again on the other side, as a packaged pair; Eagle opens into the soaring variation and then resets to begin again on the other leg before finishing.

STRETCHES (CREATING SPACE)

- Stretches the calves, hips, buttocks, lower back, shoulders, neck, wrists.
- Massages internal organs, abdomen, lymph nodes in groin and armpits.

STRENGTHENS (CREATING STEADINESS)

- Feet, ankles, legs, buttocks, core, spine, lungs, heart, entire body.
- Supports a feeling of stability, focus and balance.

PARTICULARS AND PRECAUTIONS

- Can cool or heat body, depending on practitioner.
- Aids in lymphatic drainage, digestion, detoxification, and *pranic* circulation.
- Appropriate any time of day; avoid before bedtime.
- Practice either upper body only or lower body to reduce strain (half eagle).
- Practice against a wall or seated on chair for stability.
- Avoid if acute ankle, knee, shoulder problems or extreme frailty.
- Full list of Immunity and Whole Health Benefits, page 173.

HOW TO DO IT

Breathe, connect with intention, and visualize pose before doing.

- Align the feet hip-width apart and parallel to each other.
- Bend the knees, drawing the weight of the body back toward the heels into a sustainable elevated seat.
- Lift the chest and widen evenly through the front and back of the torso, wrap the right arm underneath the left, with right fingertips into the palm of the left hand or holding onto the opposing shoulder.
- Firm the navel in toward the spine for stabilization.
- Wrap the right leg over the left leg, hugging the thighs together in the midline for support and balance.

- Align the hips and shoulders to face straight forward.
- Hug the outer hips in, squeezing the thighs and the ankles to the midline while elongating the spine.
- Hold gaze on a *drishti* or a point of focus at nose height to aid balance.
- Cultivate a slow, smooth, even breathing pattern for five breaths or whatever is sustainable.
- With intention to fly, undo the wrapping of the arms, push down into the feet, reach arms out, around, and up like the large wingspan of an eagle, transitioning into Standing Soaring Eagle Pose.

Transition into Standing Soaring Eagle Pose

URDHVA GARUDASANA
SOARING EAGLE POSE

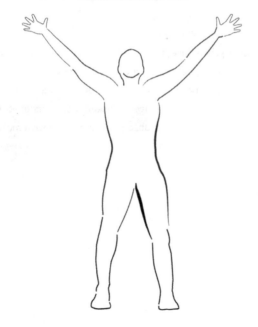

- Root down into the feet to push you up to rise tall into Soaring Eagle.
- Step the feet a leg-length distance apart while reaching arms up in a V the same width.
- Inhale and breathe deep, lifting the chest and the face to the sky.
- Stay longer than you think you should and invigorate the body and soul upwards.
- Slowly bring hands together at the chest center to stand in Mountain Pose.
- Breathe, stabilize, and reset to prepare to do the other side.

Repeat Garudasana/Eagle Pose (page 177) for the opposite leg and arm, finishing in Standing Soaring Eagle.

Complete with Mountain Pose (page 45) or Standing Forward Fold (page 54).

Drishti (DRI-shtee): When the eyes wander, our energy and focus disperses. We utilize one-pointed focus, a gazing point or drishti, to create physical and mental balance. The consistent practice of *ekagrata*, or one-pointed focus, creates the pathway to peacefulness, prolonged concentration or meditation, and the absorption state called *samadhi*, or absorption into the present moment.

DANDASANA
(DAWN-DAH-SA-NA)
STAFF POSE

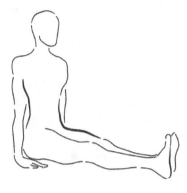

BALANCE, FOCUS, CALM ALERTNESS, RESILIENCE

A cousin of Mountain Pose, this seated posture holds the key to all of the other seated postures and supports the body in an efficient, energized way. This neutral, symmetrical position is the baseline template to which we will compare all the other seated postures. Compare and contrast to see where there may be unconscious imbalances being created in the mind and body. Mountain Pose establishes a stable, symmetrical joint and internal organ health baseline. Arms down or arms up, this pose creates balance, clarity, and intelligence in our actions and is the blueprint for physical vitality.

STRETCHES (CREATING SPACE)

- Stretches the back leg, hips, buttocks, spine
- Creates space in lower back, relieving back pain

STRENGTHENS (CREATING STEADINESS)

- Strengthens legs, spine, core
- Supports a feeling of focus and stability

PARTICULARS AND PRECAUTIONS

- Cools the body.
- Appropriate any time of day/evening.
- Can be practiced between other poses to calm and reset the system.
- Bend the knees if any strain in the low back.
- Place hands on a block to create space in the upper back.
- Avoid if you have spinal disc issues or sciatic pain.
- Full list of Immunity and Whole Health Benefits, page 173.

Start the pose with bent knees, hands on the outside of the hips, chest lifted and open, lifting the belly up from the thighs to shift the body weight forward toward the pubic bone, away from the tailbone, as preparation to go into the full straight-legged pose.

HOW TO DO IT

Breathe, connect with intention, and visualize pose before doing.

- Sitting on the floor with the legs stretched out (consider utilizing a folded blanket under the hips to support tilt of the hips, supporting the lift of the spine).
- While straightening the legs, align the heels directly in line with the frontal hip points.
- Flex the feet and press the thighs down toward the floor.
- Shift the body weight from the tailbone forward toward the pubic bone to support the natural curve of the low back. Avoid tucking the tailbone and flattening the low back curve.
- Firm the core muscles and lift the sternum up, away from the hips, to sit up tall.
- Place the hands alongside the hips on the floor, push down to help the upper body lift up.
- Hold gaze straight ahead, nose height, chin parallel to the floor.
- Breathe evenly and slowly, holding the pose for up to eight breaths.

VIRABHADRASANA 3
(VEER-A-BAH-DRAHS-AH-NA)
WARRIOR 3 POSE

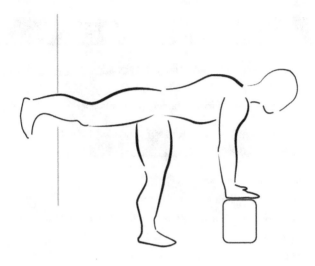

COURAGE, ENDURANCE, FOCUS, STRENGTH, PREPARATORY FOR
ACTIVE INVERSIONS

Considered to be one of the more advanced standing and balancing postures, Vira 3 builds strength, stability, and courage, all at the same time. It can be readily modified to increase focus and balance by placing the heel of the lifted leg against the wall, similar to Tabletop posture, straight back from the buttocks, parallel to the floor. Here the root name Vira truly lives up to the translation of courage, as this pose delivers an energy of fearlessness and follow-through. Consider this a preparatory pose for a more complex Supported Handstand against a wall, where we slowly, methodically step into our greatest vision of our life and highest intentions and that, let's face it, takes great courage.

STRETCHES (CREATING SPACE)

- Stretches the back leg, hips, buttocks, lower abdomen, spine, chest, shoulders
- Creates space in lower back, relieving back pain

STRENGTHENS (CREATING STEADINESS)

- Strengthens feet, legs, buttocks, outer hip, spine, core, lungs, heart, shoulders
- Supports a feeling of focus, stamina and confidence

PARTICULARS AND PRECAUTIONS

- Creates heat in the body.
- Appropriate any time, but avoid before bedtime.
- Avoid knee injury by keeping knee stacked over the ankle and pointed straight ahead.
- Press back heel to a wall and place hands on chair or blocks for balance and stability.
- Avoid if acute low back or knee problems or extreme frailty; if high blood pressure, consider placing hands on blocks, chair, or wall.
- Full list of Immunity and Whole Health Benefits, page 173.

HOW TO DO IT

Breathe, connect with intention, and visualize pose before doing.

- Utilizing a wall, measure a leg's-length distance away (more info page 187).
- Adjust as needed to align the back-leg heel to the wall with body-hip-leg in a ninety-degree or T shape.
- Consider utilizing blocks or two sturdy books directly underneath the shoulders for additional stability.

- Draw the lifted leg, hip down, into line with the standing hip to create a neutral pelvis and hip structure.
- Activate the standing leg's outer hip muscle inward and activate the core.
- Press the heel from the buttocks firmly into the wall to stabilize and energize the body.
- Elongate the spine by pulling the chest forward, creating a long line from heel to head.
- Reach out with one arm, with the palm facing the midline directly (like alternate arm leg).
- Once stable, reach the other arm forward to hold, or, if unsustainable, balance with hands on blocks/books.
- Cultivate steady and spacious; take any struggle out of the posture.
- Breathe evenly, cultivating steadiness and spaciousness.
- Bend the knees to slowly transition out of the pose and step the back foot down with the front foot.
- Stabilize in Mountain Pose, then proceed to do the other leg/side.
- Consider finishing in Standing Forward Fold page 54 or Child's Pose page 58.

ADHO MUKHA VRIKSASANA
(AH-DOH MOO-KHA VRIK-SHA-SA-NA)
SUPPORTED HANDSTAND

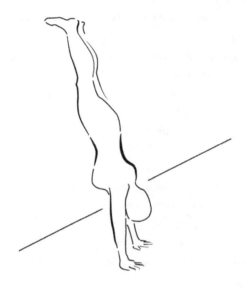

COURAGE, ENDURANCE, FOCUS, STRENGTH, CREATES SYSTEM RESET

As we move from Vira 3 posture into the more complex Supported Handstand using a wall, we are slowly, methodically stepping into our strength, endurance, resilience, and courage. This posture uses steady and skilled action to move the body upside down rather than momentum. Ideally, there is no kicking to get up and no jumping, sliding, or falling to get down. Methodically strengthen, detox, and move through fear to shift into a whole-body-focused perspective. Instead of gymnastic, consider this transition and posture a focus exercise and a *moving meditation*.

STRETCHES (CREATING SPACE)

- Stretches hands, arms, shoulders, chest, spine, buttocks, legs
- Creates space in spinal discs and lower back, relieving back pain
- Creates space in lower abdomen aiding digestion/elimination

STRENGTHENS (CREATING STEADINESS)

- Strengthens hands, arms, shoulders, core, lungs, heart, legs
- Creates stamina, confidence, focus, and feeling of courage

PARTICULARS AND PRECAUTIONS

- Creates heat in the body.
- Shifts perspective, reverses effects of gravity, aids in detoxification.
- Appropriate any time; avoid before bedtime.
- Practice alternating the leading leg stepping up to balance the body.
- If this pose is not sustainable, practice Legs Up the Wall in its place, page 211.
- Avoid if wrist or shoulder injury, frailty, high blood pressure, glaucoma, history of stroke, or acute fear.
- Full list of Immunity and Whole Health Benefits, page 173.

Measurement of a Leg's Distance Tip: A helpful way to measure the leg's distance is to sit in Staff Pose (image page 181), sit with the back of the hips firmly pressed to the wall with the legs extended straight out with heels flexed. Measure where the heels of the feet align on the floor, as that is where the heels will go for Warrior 3, or the root of the hands for Downward-Facing Dog for Supported Handstand. If you have a yoga block or some kind of visual marker, place it in line with the heels before the transition from Staff Pose to the next pose.

HOW TO DO IT

Breathe, connect with intention, and visualize pose before doing.

- Measure the length of the legs in Staff Pose (as just described on page 187) and note where the heels align.
- Place the root of the hands where the heels of the feet were to create Downward-Facing Dog (page 60).
- Place heel of the feet at the meeting of the wall and floor.

- *Note this Down Dog will feel shorter than the regular length that was practiced earlier in the book.*
- Spread the fingers evenly and anchor the weight into the thumb and index finger.
- Firm the forearms and the outer upper arms gently toward each other to stabilize the shoulders.
- Stack the shoulders directly over the wrists, look slightly forward to draw the upper back in toward chest.
- Once stabilized, step one foot around two feet, or sustainably a quarter of the way, up the wall, pressing strongly into the foot to begin to leverage the body in a slight inversion. *This is a great place to stay and step back down to repeat on the other leg. Continue to repeat to build strength and confidence.*
- If proceeding, step one foot up again onto the wall, pressing to lift the body.
- Step with other leg, walking all the way up the wall into a supported handstand.
- Press down into the hands and rebound through the rest of body and legs.
- Firm the outer upper arms toward each other to stabilize the shoulder joints.
- Engage the legs and pull up through the body.
- Continue to lengthen up through side waist so the torso is even on all sides.
- Breathe, holding as long as steady, balanced, and relaxed simultaneously.
- Do not over-hold or cultivate struggle!
- Save energy and stability to carefully, slowly step, in control, down the wall to Child's Pose.

BENEFITS OF INVERTING

Inverting the body reverses gravitational pressure, which reduces stress on the spinal column. It aids breathing, circulation, digestion, lymphatic drainage, and veins returning blood to the heart, which all aids in detoxification and immune function. Increased blood circulation can have benefit on cognitive function and may relieve headaches. Inverting can be strength, balance, and confidence building, as well as calming and releasing. Literally and figuratively, it can help shift the world upside down to expand our view and open opportunities.

ARDHA MATSYENDRASANA
ARD-AH MAHT-SEE-EN-DRAH-SA-NA)
SEATED TWIST POSE

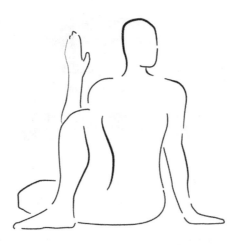

BALANCE, FOCUS, RELEASE, HIP OPENER, SPINAL ROTATION

This is an accessible version of a pose that has many variations. As with other spinal twists, there is a detoxification and massaging effect with the posture. Wonderful for preparing for the more subtle practices of pranayama and meditation, as it holds the added benefit of drawing energy and awareness to the axial line in the center of the body, deepening focus and gathering of our attention.

Similar to setting up Staff Pose, sit toward the front top of one or two folded blankets or bath towels to elevate the hips and tilt the hips slightly forward to take strain out of the low back and spine. Align the sitting bones toward the end of the blanket fold, versus in the middle of the pile, to aid in the tilt forward guiding the weight of the body toward the pubic bone and away from the tailbone.

STRETCHES (CREATING SPACE)

- Stretches the outer hip, buttocks, spine, chest, shoulders
- Creates space in lower back, relieving back pain
- Massages internal organs and abdomen

STRENGTHENS (CREATING STEADINESS)

- Strengthens legs, spine, core, and upper back
- Supports a feeling of focus, stability, and calmness

PARTICULARS AND PRECAUTIONS

- Cools the body.
- Appropriate any time day/evening.
- Sit forward on folded blanket to support spine, lift and tilt hips slightly forward.
- Place back hand on a block to lift chest, creating space in the upper back.
- Avoid if you have knee issues, spinal disc issues, or sciatic pain.
- Full list of Immunity and Whole Health Benefits, page 173.

HOW TO DO IT

Breathe, connect with intention, and visualize pose before doing.

- Starting in Staff Pose, bend and bring one of the legs up toward the chest.
- As you make space for the other leg to bend, drawing the heel toward the outside of the other hip.
- Bring the first leg over the bent one near the hip, creating a semi-pretzel twist of the legs.
- Align the sitting bones on the floor to be as even as possible, as the lifted leg hip and buttock bone may lift.

- Draw the lifted hip down will aid in supporting space of the low back and spinal discs.
- As with Staff Pose, continue to shift the weight of the body off of the tailbone and forward toward the pubic bone, cultivating the low back curve, versus tucking the tailbone to flatten the curve.
- Lift through the spine to create as much length then firm the low belly to begin to twist the upper back.
- Turn the chest toward the side of the lifted leg which is in toward the body.
- Use the back arm to help maintain the spinal lift.
- Deepen the twist with use of the front hand, arm, or elbow.
- Inhale, lengthen the spine; exhale, deepen the twist.
- Anchor the hips, turn from the chest, and allow the head to go last, following the movement of chest.
- Repeat with the opposite leg in front crossed over the top, twisting the other way.
- Return to Staff Pose when complete.
- Remain on blanket lift and proceed to Janu Shirshasana/Head-to-Knee Pose.

JANU SHIRSHASANA
(JON-OO SHEER-SHA-SAH-NA)
HEAD-TO-KNEE POSE

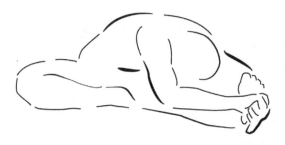

BALANCE, FOCUS, CALM ALERTNESS, SURRENDER

A forward fold and gentle twist massage for the lower abdominal cavity, this pose is quieting and a gathering of attention for greater focus. The pose guides us to go deeper into ourselves, breath by breath, layer by layer, until we draw into the essential core of pure life.

STRETCHES (CREATING SPACE)

- Stretches the outer hip, back of leg, buttocks, spine, chest, shoulders
- Creates space in lower back, relieving back pain
- Massages internal organs and abdomen

STRENGTHENS (CREATING STEADINESS)

- Strengthens legs, spine, core and upper back
- Supports a feeling of focus, stability, and calmness

- Cools the body.
- Relieves back pain when both sides of the pelvis remain even and neutral.
- Appropriate any time day/evening.
- Sit forward on folded blanket to support spine, lift and tilt hips slightly forward.
- Utilize strap over the extended leg foot or bend the knee to lengthen the spine.
- Avoid if you have knee issues, spinal disc issues, or sciatic pain.
- Full list of Immunity and Whole Health Benefits, page 173.

HOW TO DO IT

Breathe, connect with intention, and visualize pose before doing.

- Start out sitting on a blanket lift in Staff Pose.
- Bend one knee, rotate the upper leg bone outward to place foot into the opposite inner thigh area.
- Avoid putting pressure on the knee joint.
- Even out the sitting bones on the floor or blankets.
- Shift the body weight forward, off of the tailbone, toward the pubic bone, to encourage low back curve.
- Lift pelvic floor and lower abdomen to lift up through the spine, lifting the sternum away from the waist.
- Inhale, elongate spine; exhale, micro twist toward the leg to seal the belly lift in place.
- Keep the low belly lifted and turn the chest toward the extended straight leg.
- Hinge from the hips with the front of the torso stretching (avoid rounding the upper back).
- Hold the bottom of the extended foot, with toe lock (info following page 194) or strap.

- Avoid rounding, utilize a strap or towel to add extension to the arms for spinal length.
- Lengthen all sides of the waist evenly as you pull the sternum away from the navel.
- Broaden through the chest, draw the shoulders away from the ears, lengthen evenly through neck.
- Gaze to the big toe.
- Breathe evenly, cultivating steady and spacious sustainable hold.
- Slowly release and return to Staff Pose to reset.
- Repeat on the other side, same quality and duration.
- After both sides, return back to Staff Pose to feel, harmonize, and reflect.

Creating a Toe Lock: Hook the index and middle finger around the big toe is considered a classic toe lock or sometimes referred to as a Yogic Toe Lock, to be done with flexed feet and stable toe base, or on the metatarsals. Press through the big toe mound as you guide the pinky toes back toward the body. This can be used on standing and seated forward folds.

POSES FOR FREEDOM

PURVOTTANASANA
(PURR-VOH-TA-NA-SA-NA)
REVERSE TABLETOP

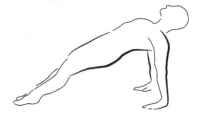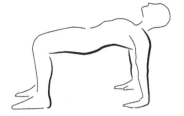

COURAGE, PURPOSE, EXPRESSION, STRENGTH-BUILDING ENERGIZER

Mindfully turning the body inside out to encourage clearing, forward movement, and release. Opening the body in back bending is energizing, and this posture also incorporates direct expansion through the throat, thyroid, and thymus gland region, directly stimulating breath, expression, immunity, and hormone function.

STRETCHES (CREATING SPACE)

- Front of legs, abdomen, chest, spine, shoulders, throat, wrists and hands
- Creates space in the entire front body

STRENGTHENS (CREATING STEADINESS)

- Feet, ankles, legs, buttocks, core, spine, shoulders, wrists, and hands
- Invigorates lungs, heart, and whole body

PARTICULARS AND PRECAUTIONS

- Creates heat in the body.
- Stimulates the throat, thyroid, and thymus gland.

- Avoid evening or before bedtime.
- Practice half version with knees bent, feet on the floor, if full is unsustainable.
- Avoid if wrist, shoulder, low back, groin, or neck issues, or if frail.
- Full list of Immunity and Whole Health Benefits, page 173.

HOW TO DO IT

Breathe, connect with intention, and visualize pose before doing.

- Sitting on the floor, with the legs hip-width apart, knees bent, stacked over the ankles.
- Align the hands with fingers pointing toward the hips, behind the body, shoulder-width apart.
- Press through the feet and hands to lift the hips in line with the chest and shoulders.
- Firm the belly to support the spine, and lengthen the neck, keeping the head in line with the shoulders.
- Spin the inner thighs down toward the floor as you lengthen the buttocks toward the knees, creating space for the low back.
- If you feel stable and are breathing smoothly, proceed to the full straight-leg pose.
- Straighten one leg at a time until the heels are the new anchor of the pose.
- Firm the abdomen and support the head so there is no strain on the neck.
- Press the heels down as you lift the hips in line with the chest to open the front body.
- Cultivate smooth, even, balanced breaths, a minimum of three breaths, a maximum of eight.
- Soften the knees to undo the pose.
- Mindfully walk the feet back, bending the knees to stack over the ankles.
- Slowly lower the buttocks back to the floor.
- Stabilize the body and breath to reset.
- Proceed to supine (on the back) for Thread the Needle Pose.

SUPTA KAPOTANASANA

SUPINE PIGEON, THREAD THE NEEDLE

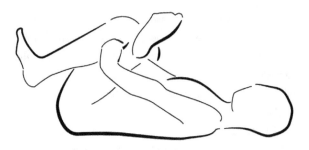

HIP-OPENING, LOW BACK RELEASE, FOCUS, CALMING

This hip opener and low back release posture can be adapted into many variations, including seated on a chair. It can help relieve pressure on the sciatic nerve and creates space for the low back when the hips are drawn down evenly on both sides. The benefits of this posture are amplified with the hips in neutral, when the lifted side hip isn't hiked up toward the shoulder. Give special attention to this balance, and this posture will be a good friend.

STRETCHES (CREATING SPACE)

- Stretches the outer hip, back of leg, buttocks, spine, chest, shoulders
- Creates space in lower back, relieving back pain
- Massages internal organs and abdomen

STRENGTHENS (CREATING STEADINESS)

- Strengthens legs, spine, core, and upper back
- Supports a feeling of focus, stability, and calmness

PARTICULARS AND PRECAUTIONS

- Cools the body.
- Relieves back pain when both sides of the pelvis remain even and neutral.
- Appropriate any time of day/evening.
- Can be practiced seated in an upright proper seat on a chair.
- Flex the foot to stabilize the ankle to avoid sickling and stretching the ankle.
- Utilize strap behind leg, creating length for arms, to allow for proper spinal alignment.
- Avoid if you have knee, spinal disc, shoulder, or neck issues.
- Full list of Immunity and Whole Health Benefits, page 173.

HOW TO DO IT

Breathe, connect with intention, and visualize pose before doing.

- Recline supine (on the back), feet on the floor, parallel to each other with knees stacked over the heels.
- Lengthen through the spine, creating symmetry in the body.
- Move the upper back in to support the natural curve of the neck.
- Draw the right thigh into the chest, keeping the knee bent with foot flexed, rotate the thigh outward from the body, and cross the ankle or shin over the left thigh.
- Draw the right lifted hip down on an even plane with the left, so the low back and sacral area is in symmetry or neutral position. (The therapeutic application of this posture is based in the back of the hips being even to support a steady and spacious low back.)
- If this feels like an intense stretch, stay and breathe here as your stopping point.
- Deepen the stretch by drawing the leg structure upright, stacking the left knee over the frontal hip points.
- Continue to rotate at the right leg in the hip socket, gently stretching the leg out to the side.

- Keep the ankle flexed so there is no unintentional stretch through the ankle.
- Either with the hands, or threading a strap or belt, thread through the center gap of the legs to bind for leverage behind the left thigh, as in "threading the needle."
- Anchor the back of the shoulders and head to the mat, continuing to draw the lifted hip down evenly.
- Breathe evenly and fully until ready to proceed to the other side at same quality and duration.
- Complete by drawing knees into the chest (page 134) and breathe a series of Full Complete Breaths (page 77).
- Roll to the side in fetal position, supporting the head with bottom arm, to hold for a few breaths before coming upright.

Starting on the right side supports elimination, as it gives the ascending colon a massage, and then practice on the left side giving the descending colon a massage. Consider practicing right leg first, then proceed to the left leg.

PASCHIMOTTANASANA
(PAH-SHEE-MOH-TA-NAH-SA-NA)
SEATED FORWARD FOLD

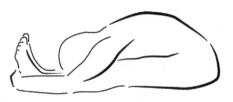

BALANCE, FOCUS, CALM, SURRENDER

Often referred to as West Side Stretch, as the sun goes down in the west and so does our asana practice. Our practice begins to cool and approach its close with this seated forward fold. We honor all that has come before, and the process of becoming. This is a complex forward fold for a stiffer body, as it relies on deep and subtle actions inside the pelvis and abdomen to create the fold. If you over effort it or force it with lack of understanding, the spine will round, with little benefit and plenty of risk. The magic of the pose is dependent on an inner clarity and trust of the process to get there. The legs anchor the posture, and the pelvis is the moving part; the spine just follows in line with the movement of the pelvis. As you are sitting on the pelvis with gravity pulling it down, it takes a huge amount of inner fortitude to shift the seemingly unmovable. The pose represents bigger life elements at work; anchor into the pelvis or earth, draw up power or fire from the belly, elongate and lead humbly from the heart. We can't skip any step of this journey, breath by breath, acceptance by acceptance, and we arrive to experience the beautiful sunset.

STRETCHES (CREATING SPACE)

- Massages internal organs and abdomen

STRENGTHENS (CREATING STEADINESS)

- Front of hip, legs, core, and spine
- Supports a feeling of stability and calmness

- Cools and calms the body.
- Increases posterior lung expansion and air circulation.
- Bend the knees, utilize a strap over balls of the feet to extend the arms, and sit up on folded blankets if any strain in the low back.
- Avoid if you have spinal disc issues, hiatal hernia, sciatic pain, or hamstring injury.
- Full list of Immunity and Whole Health Benefits, page 173.

HOW TO DO IT

Breathe, connect with intention, and visualize pose before doing.

- Start in Staff Pose with bent knees.
- Shift the body weight from the tailbone forward toward the pubic bone to support the natural curve of the low back.
- Avoid tucking the tailbone and flattening the low back curve.
- Straighten the legs.
- Align the heels directly in line with hips, feet flexed, pressing the thighs down toward the floor.
- Lift the sternum up away from the hips to sit up tall, inspire stretch of the front body.
- Use a strap over the balls of the feet or utilize the hands in a classic toe lock over big toes if using hands.
- Continue to press down through the upper leg bones, keeping the legs in neutral, not rolling them out or in, while lifting long through low belly up the spine, hinge from the hips to bring the lower belly close to the thighs while avoiding rounding the upper back.
- Continue elongating the front body as you hold at the sustainable amount of stretch for the body; avoid rounding the spin and tucking the chin.
- Cultivate a balance of steady slow stretching with a sense of spacious relaxation.
- Breathe evenly and slowly and hold a soft gaze on the big toes.
- Release the bind of strap or hands and proceed to a reclined supine position.

SUPTA PADANGUSTHASANA
(SOOP-TA PAH-DAHN-GOOSH-STAH-SA-NA)
RECLINED HAND TO FOOT (STRAP TO FOOT)

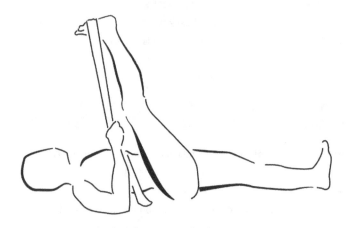

LOW BACK RELEASE, FOCUS, STABILITY, CALM

This hamstring stretch and low back release posture can be adapted into many variations, including a supine twist. Similar to Supine Pigeon, this posture can help relieve pressure on the sciatic nerve and creates space for the low back when the hips are drawn down evenly on both sides. Again, the benefits of this posture are amplified with the hips in neutral when the lifted side hip isn't hiked up toward the shoulder. This posture is so much more than a stretch; it is balm to the spine and deeply calming to the mind.

STRETCHES (CREATING SPACE)

- Back of legs, low back, spine, shoulders, arms, and lungs
- Massages internal organs and abdomen

STRENGTHENS (CREATING STEADINESS)

- Strengthens feet, legs, core, spine
- Supports a feeling of balance, stability, and calmness

PARTICULARS AND PRECAUTIONS

- Cools and calms the body.
- Increases posterior lung expansion and air circulation.
- Appropriate any time or day/evening.
- Can be practiced between other poses to calm and reset the system.
- Bend the knee, utilize a strap over balls of the foot to extend the arms to relieve strain in the low back.
- Avoid if you have spinal disc issues, hiatal hernia, sciatic pain, or hamstring injury.
- Full list of Immunity and Whole Health Benefits, page 173.

HOW TO DO IT

Breathe, connect with intention, and visualize pose before doing.

- Lying supine on the back, feet on the floor, parallel to each other, with knees stacked over the heels.
- Lengthen through the spine, creating symmetry in the body, while drawing the upper back in to support the natural curve of the neck.
- Draw the right thigh into the chest, with knee bent, foot flexed, and wrap a strap or belt around ball of the foot.
- With strap in hand, draw the elbows down to the side of the torso, anchored to the floor.
- Stabilize the wrists (straight without sickling) and press the elbows into the floor, hugging close to the body.
- Draw the right lifted hip down on an even plane with the left, so the low back and sacral area is in symmetry or neutral position. *Similar to Thread the Needle Pose, part of the therapeutic application of*

this posture is based in the back of the hips being even to support a steady and spacious low back.

- *If there is any discomfort in the low back, keep the left foot on the floor and work to straighten the right leg while drawing the right back of the hip down even with the left.*

- Straighten the opposite leg; anchor buttocks and thigh bone toward the floor.

- Keeping the leg in neutral (not turned out or in), anchor the left leg to the floor.

- Draw the right leg closer to the abdomen.

- Keep the back of the shoulders, the head, and the extended leg to the mat.

- Breathe deeply, cultivating steady and spacious.

- Proceed to repeat on the other side with equal quality and duration.

- When both sides are complete with same quality and length of hold, draw both thighs into the chest, creating Knees To Chest Pose (page 134) for a few breaths before proceeding to Bound Plough Pose (omit Bound Plough Pose if there is any history of neck injury).

Utilize a strap or belt over the ball of the lifted foot rather than using the hand in a classic big toe lock. Consider only doing the toe lock if the back of the shoulder and head remain rooted on the floor, draw the upper back in to support the neck curve and draw the tailbone down, supporting the low back curve.

BADDHA HALASANA
(BAH-DAH HAH-LAH-SA-NA)
BOUND PLOUGH POSE

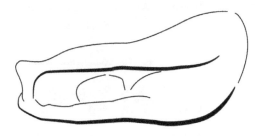

CALM, RELEASE, SURRENDER, THYROID AND THYMUS MASSAGE

My dear mother, Nunna to my boys, used to do this pose with them on the floor when they were little and joyfully call "Let's do piggies in the air pose!" This particular version cultivates the same sweet release and sentiment, yet we hold the piggies (ahem, feet/big toes) to create a cradle to protect the neck from strain and being overstretched. Therefore, holding the feet is important here, and when not utilizing the bind, it is recommended to practice with a couple of folded blankets under the upper back and shoulders to protect the neck.

STRETCHES (CREATING SPACE)

- Back of legs, low back, spine, shoulders, arms, neck and lungs
- Massages internal organs, abdomen, and throat

STRENGTHENS (CREATING STEADINESS)

- Strengthens feet, legs, core, spine
- Supports a feeling of balance, stability, and calmness

PARTICULARS AND PRECAUTIONS

- Cools and calms the body.
- Massages thyroid and thymus glands in the throat.
- Increases posterior lung expansion and air circulation.
- Appropriate any time of day/evening.
- Avoid if history of neck injury, spinal disc issues, hiatal hernia, sciatic pain, or hamstring injury.
- Full list of Immunity and Whole Health Benefits, page 173.

HOW TO DO IT

Breathe, connect with intention, and visualize pose before doing.

- Align the feet hip-width apart and parallel to each other.
- Reclining supine on the back, draw the thighs into the chest similar to Knees to Chest (page 134).
- Place hands on the back of the thighs and straighten the legs, pressing the heels toward the sky.
- If there is any pressure or discomfort in the low back or spine, stay here, bend the knees and repeat the straightening of the legs as the posture; do not proceed to the next phase of Bound Plough.
- Reach for the feet and create a toe lock with both hands and feet (toe lock information on page 194).
- Draw the shoulders back down toward the floor and support the neck curve staying intact.
- Firm the belly, lift the leg structure over the head until the feet (still bound by the hands in the toe lock) meet the floor.
- If there is any discomfort, please slowly undo, bringing the hips and legs back down to the floor.
- Stabilize and deepen by pressing tops of bound toes to floor behind the head.
- Keep the head and neck straight, no rotation to either side.
- Breathe smoothly and evenly, cultivating steady and spacious.

Note: the arms over the head create a cushion for the discs in the neck and delicate spinal column. Do not practice this position without the arms up over head, unless with a seasoned yoga teacher to guide for support of spinal safety.

- Release posture by bending the knees and lowering the hips back down.
- Undo the toe lock and hug the thighs into the chest to release and reset.
- Slowly lower the feet to the floor to rest, feel effects before proceeding to next posture.

POSES FOR INTEGRATION

SUPTA BADDHA KONASANA
(SOOP-TA BAH-DAH KOH-NA-SA-NA)
RECLINED BOUND ANGLE

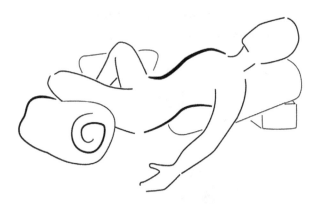

CALM, SURRENDER, LUNG EXPANSION, BELLY RELEASE

Here the legs are relaxed, open, like the wings of a butterfly. There is no effort, strain, or stretch within the opening of the legs. The blankets or pillows placed under the thighs are to stop any strain or stretch, creating a bowl of sorts within the space of the legs and belly. Fill that bowl with breath, nourishment, and contentment.

STRETCHES (CREATING SPACE)

- Outer hips, inner groin, lower back, spine, chest, shoulders, throat
- Creates space for internal organs, abdomen, lungs, and throat

STRENGTHENS (CREATING STEADINESS)

- Strengthens through restoration of immune, nervous, and endocrine systems
- Supports a feeling of balance, stability, calmness, and renewal

PARTICULARS AND PRECAUTIONS

- Cools and calms the body.
- Appropriate any time or day/evening.
- Consider this a posture for foundational pranayama (breathing) practices.
- Add an eye pillow, rolled towel, or dark covering for the eyes to relax and release of the ocular nerves.
- For low back strain, bend the knees to place feet on the floor.
- For neck strain, add a one- to two-inch folded flat low blanket under the neck and head.
- Keep the body warm. Cover feet and body with a blanket if the temperature is cool.
- Add a blanket spread underneath the body if the floor is cool.
- Avoid or modify for low back, groin, or neck issues.
- Full list of Immunity and Whole Health Benefits, page 173.

HOW TO DO IT

Breathe, connect with intention, and visualize pose before doing.

- Use a blanket or bolster to create a spine-length roll to support the spine.
- Have additional blankets or blocks in easy reach as you recline.
- Sit with buttocks on the floor and lie back on blanket roll.
- Adjust the blanket roll to support the low back and all along the spine up to the neck and head.
- Do not let the head drop back unsupported; utilize another prop to support if necessary.

- Keep the feet on the floor with the knees bent to stabilize the spine.
- Create symmetry in the body and steadiness in the breath.
- Once stable in body and breath, rotate the thighs outward externally to bring the soles of the feet together, creating a diamond shape.
- Place an even support under each thigh, just above the knee joint. Two blocks, two books, or two rolled bath towels are great for this.
- Use the supports to take all the stretch out of the groin.
- Create space through the abdomen and groin pit area without putting any strain on the body. When the body is being stretched, there is a certain amount of stimulus on the nervous system and the body is on alert.
- Support the thighs so the body fully relaxes, and the longevity functions of the body are supported.
- Practice Full Complete Breaths or Expansive Three-Part Inhalations here.
- Deepen into a gentle opening of the breath and relaxation.
- To transition out of the pose, slowly bring the knees back up and feet onto the floor.
- Stay with feet on the floor for a series of slow acclimating breaths.
- Once steady, slowly, and gently roll to the left side.
- Stay on the left side to restore until ready to slowly transition upright to seated meditation or Corpse Pose.

VIPARITA KARANI
(VIP-AH-REE-TAH KAH-RAH-NEE)
LEGS UP THE WALL OR WATERFALL POSE

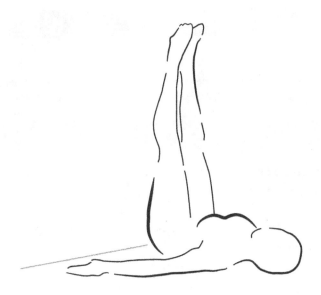

RESTORATIVE, CLEARING, CALMING, SUPPORTS SLEEP

Restore the whole being through this passive inversion. Here we practice the most basic and easy no-prop wall-support version of Viparita Karani. This posture has been touted for a long list of benefits and is shared with the key yoga wisdom texts of *Hatha Yoga Pradipika*, *Gheranda Samhita*, and *Shiva Samhita*. In this reversal of our doing, passively lifting the legs above the heart, we shift our body's flow as well as creating an opportunity to shift our inner perspective. The key to this posture is passive release and receptivity in the belly as the waterfall of *pranic* energy comes down the legs, pools there in the belly, overflows up over the heart, over the throat, and clears the third-eye inner visionary center to then continue over the crown of the head into universal connection.

STRETCHES (CREATING SPACE)

- Back of the legs, spine, chest, and shoulders
- Creates space for internal organs, abdomen, lungs, and throat

STRENGTHENS (CREATING STEADINESS)

- Strengthens through restoration of immune, nervous, and endocrine systems
- Supports a feeling of balance, stability, calmness, and renewal

PARTICULARS AND PRECAUTIONS

- Cools and calms the body.
- Supports circadian rhythm and sleep.
- Reduces edema and fluid swelling in feet/legs.
- Aids in blood detoxification by aiding the veins returning blood to the heart.
- Appropriate any time of day/evening.
- Chair, edge of a bed, etc., can be used in place of a wall.
- Add an eye pillow, rolled towel, or dark covering for the eyes to relax and release of the ocular nerves.
- For neck strain, add a one- to two-inch folded flat low blanket under the neck and head.
- Avoid or modify for low back, hamstring, or neck issues.
- Full list of Immunity and Whole Health Benefits, page 173.

HOW TO DO IT

Breathe, connect with intention, and visualize pose before doing.

- Utilizing a wall or similar, start reclined on the floor in a fetal position on one side.

- Align the buttocks about six to eight inches away from the wall and slowly, while shifting on to the back, stretch one leg onto the wall, then the other, to have both the legs up the wall.
- Shift the hips and buttocks so that the low back curve is intact.
- Lengthen tailbone down toward floor, avoiding letting it lift up the wall.
- Find the sweet spot where the tailbone is down and there is no pull on the back of the legs and low back.
- Once aligned, create symmetry through both sides of the body.
- Draw the shoulder blades in toward the chest to widen across the chest and collarbones.
- Gently adjust the chin to support the natural neck curve, bringing the chin in line with the shoulders, neither jutted up toward the ceiling nor tucked down toward the collarbones.
- Allow the body to settle, relaxing into a passive restorative state.
- Practice Full Complete Breaths or Expansive Three-Part Inhalations here.
- Deepen into a gentle opening of the breath and relaxation.
- Hold up to five minutes.
- Firm the low belly and bend the knees into the chest to roll to the left side to transition out of the pose.
- Once on the left side of the body, support the head with the bottom arm to breathe, feel, and reflect before slowly coming upright to a seated position for meditation, or recline for Shavasana/Corpse Pose or sleep.

SHAVASANA
(SHAH-VAH-SAH-NA)
CORPSE POSE

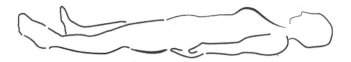

CALM, SURRENDER, LUNG EXPANSION, BELLY RELEASE

"Shavasana: Just do it," the official slogan of yoga teachers everywhere. This humble yet significant posture is the one that often gets overlooked and is the one that many of us need the most. This restorative posture helps reset the nervous system, activating the parasympathetic rest/digest response that creates a cascade of whole health benefits. This deep activation of this relaxation response slows our heart rate, blood pressure, decreases inflammation and stress hormones, supports hormone balance, aids in digestion, and boosts immune function.

STRETCHES (CREATING SPACE)

- Whole body
- Creates space for internal organs, abdomen, lungs, and throat

STRENGTHENS (CREATING STEADINESS)

- Strengthens through restoration of immune, nervous, and endocrine systems
- Supports a feeling of balance, stability, calmness, and renewal

- Cools and calms the body.
- Slows brain waves to calm the system.
- Appropriate any time or day/evening.
- Practice on the belly, head turned to the side, when processing grief or anxiety.
- Add an eye pillow, rolled towel, or dark covering for the eyes to relax and release of the ocular nerves.
- For low back strain, place rolled blanket or pillow under the knees.
- For neck strain, add a one- to two-inch folded flat low blanket under the neck and head.
- Keep the body warm. Cover feet, and add a blanket under and over the body if cool.
- Full list of Immunity and Whole Health Benefits, page 173.

TWENTY-ONE-DAY SHAVASANA/CORPSE POSE PRACTICE INSPIRATION

With the intention of making healing a priority, resetting the nervous system from a chronic overdrive response, join me in the Twenty-One-Day Shavasana/Corpse Pose Practice. It is possibly the most important practice of this entire chapter, arguably the entire book.

Each day—maybe midafternoon, as it may be an ideal time between two and four o'clock when your energy may wane, or any time you think is right—consider moving the spine gently in all directions and then recline for a minimum of five minutes, up to twenty minutes. Do it each day, for twenty-one days *and hopefully beyond.*

It's okay if you miss a day, "oh well," make it a priority the next day. Remember to make the body and mind comfortable by making sure you are warm enough and that the low back and neck are stable, maybe adding a small pillow under the knees and a flat blanket fold under the neck.

I can feel the relaxation already. What do you say? I'll meet you there. Keep a journal log and note the benefits. Write to me and let me know how it went.

Breathe, connect with intention, and visualize pose before doing.

- Utilize a space where you can maintain stillness and calm.
- Recline supine on the back and create symmetry in the body (both sides are the same).
- Make any adjustments, including adding props as needed, so that the spinal column is in its natural curves and there is little effort in the body.
- Gently release the legs to create space in the low back.
- Gently draw the shoulder blades in toward the chest to widen across the chest and collarbones.
- Gently adjust the chin to support the natural neck curve, bringing the chin in line with the shoulders, neither jutted up toward the ceiling nor tucked down toward the collarbones.
- Make any final micro-adjustments as needed in preparation for stillness.
- Allow the body to settle, relaxing into a passive restorative state.
- Begin to bring awareness to the exhalation and very gently extend the exhalation longer than the inhalation.
- Without concern for ratio or timing, continue to subtly extend the exhalation until the awareness and the body has a feeling of total relaxation and dissolve.
- Hold for five to twenty minutes.
- To transition out of the pose, press the tongue into the roof of the mouth and gently over the front teeth; feel into the fingers and toes.
- Slowly beginning to stretch and move, firm the low belly and bend the knees into the chest to roll to the left side to transition out of the pose.
- Once on the left side of the body, support the head with the bottom arm to breathe, feel, and reflect before slowly coming upright to a seated position for meditation, or recline for Shavasana/Corpse Pose or sleep.

CHAPTER 11

PRANAYAMAS AND MEDITATIONS FOR INTEGRATION

Building on clarity and helpful detoxification practices, we are now growing assimilation of what is nourishing and helpful. Here, we bring it together in targeted breathing tools of balance, focus, freedom, and whole health integration.

As with any positive habit we hope to integrate to become a part of us, these tools are simple and easy to repeat, and they feel good to do. It gives us a perfect feedback loop to positively transform from the inside out, one breath and intention at a time.

Note of caution for the practices included in this chapter: though they are helpful and generally safe for most practitioners, yet they do build on the previous tools and strengths of Parts I and II and call for accumulative understanding, endurance, and restraint. Remember that less is more here, and if you have any sense of dizziness or loss of general steadiness, to stop the practice and restabilize. Breathing exercises are never to be done in an agitated or reactive state. Certain practices (which will be notated specifically in the Precautions and Particulars section) are not recommended for those who suffer from acute high/low blood pressure, history of stroke, diagnosed schizophrenia, or acute trauma. Those practices can be aggravating to the above conditions and should only be practiced with the loving care of an experienced yoga teacher and professional support.

Similar to Chapter 10 with the postures, I have sub-categorized the practices in this chapter as especially enhancing focus, freedom, and whole health integration. Of course, all of these exercises are a fantastic boost to the immune system and whole health.

IMMUNITY AND WHOLE HEALTH BENEFITS OF THE FOLLOWING EXERCISES

- Increase oxygen intake and decrease carbon dioxide/debris/stale air.
- Increases blood oxygen and lymphatic and digestive circulation.
- Increases lung/diaphragm strength and elasticity.
- Decreases stress overdrive functions, heart rate, blood pressure, and inflammation.
- Stimulates the vagus nerve, activating the rest/digest Response (description on page 66).
- Mindful repetitions support the slowing of brain waves and calming the mind.
- Cultivates present-moment awareness, supporting focus, concentration, mental/emotional balance.
- Supports self-regulation, resilience, endurance, and whole-system balance.
- Reduces anxiety, depression, fatigue, brain fog, and feelings of overwhelm.
- With intention, focuses the Reticular Activating System (RAS) on positive healing outcome.
- Activates vital energy currents in the body, increasing health, vitality, and radiance.

PRACTICES FOR FOCUS

A REVISIT OF BREATH RATIOS

1:1 is a generic ratio of inhalation to exhalation.

4:4 is a 4-count inhalation to a 4-count exhalation.

When retentions or pauses are used, the ratio looks like this: **1:1:1:1**

For example, in the Box Breathing Practice below, we have a 5:5:5:5 breath ratio.

5-count inhalation

to

5-count retention at the top of the inhalation, holding the breath in.

to

5-count exhalation

to

5-count retention at the bottom of the exhalation, holding the breath out.

5:5:5:5 SAMA VRITTI
(SAH-MA VREE-TEE)
BOX BREATHING

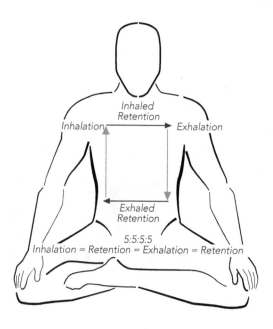

CALMING, BALANCING, FOCUSING, SUPPORTS CREATIVITY

A basic recipe for whole-system balance, box breathing is true to its name, as it involves equal lengths and portions of breathing on all sides. Inhale, connect to inspiration, hold, sustain, be nourished, exhale clear out, hold the breath, and release into harmony. There is a reason box breathing is utilized by the Navy SEALS in training, as it is a potent tool for focus, clarity, and power. Create a sustainable 5-count inhalation, 5-count gentle hold or retention at the top of the inhalation, holding the breath in, 5-count exhalation, and 5-count gentle hold or retention at the bottom of the exhalation, holding the breath out. If that feels strained, reduce to 4:4:4:4, or to what can be sustained.

- Cultivates focus, balance, relaxation into meditative state.
- Appropriate any time of day/evening.
- Cultivate sustainable ratio lengths, never forcing or straining.

HOW TO DO IT

Stabilize body, elongate spine, cultivating balance; sitting or reclined position can be used.

- Create *Gyana Mudra/*Wisdom Hand Seal in both hands (see page 90).
- Exhale the breath completely out and pause it for a moment.
- Inhale through the nose for a slow 5-count and then pause at the top of the inhale to retain the breath.
- Retain and hold the inhalation in for 5 counts, or equal to the inhalation.
- Exhale smoothly out for 5 counts and pause at the bottom of the exhalation.
- Retain and hold the exhalation out for 5 counts, or equal to all the other breath lengths.
- Continue to cultivate 5-count inhalation; 5-count hold; 5-count exhalation; 5-count hold.
- Repeat for three rounds: if sustainable and enjoyable, repeat for another eight rounds.
- Sit quietly for a minimum of one minute, observing how you feel, and to restore.
- Consider proceeding to one of the meditations shared in this book or to take Shavasana/Corpse Pose.

ANULOMA VILOMA
(AH-NOO-LOHM-AH VEE-LOHM-AH)

AND

NADI SHODHANAM
(NAH-DEE SHOH-DHA-NAHM)

ALTERNATE NOSTRIL BREATHING (WITHOUT AND WITH BREATH RETENTIONS)

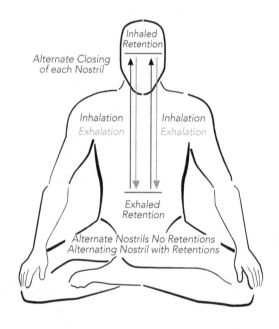

Inhaled Retention

Alternate Closing of each Nostril

Inhalation
Exhalation

Inhalation
Exhalation

Exhaled Retention

Alternate Nostrils No Retentions
Alternating Nostril with Retentions

BALANCE, FOCUS, CALM, ENHANCES COGNITIVE FUNCTION

This balancing breath has many variations and can be categorized as a kriya or cleansing technique as well as a pranayama breathing technique. It is normal and natural for the nostrils to shift in dominance depending on the time of day. Bringing the nostrils to balance using alternate nostril breathing has been shown in multiple studies to reduce blood pressure, increase mental focus, and support greater feelings of well-being. The active dominant nostril is the one with more airflow, and the passive nondominant one will have little to none.

Each nostril also coincides with an energy channel or *nadi*, and when we concentrate breath and energy through that channel, it can activate, calm, and balance activity in that brain hemisphere. The breath balances between the two nostrils in meditation, in deep relaxation, or naturally about every eighty-eight minutes. When we alternate the nostrils, it helps bring the hemispheres to balance, bringing harmony, calm, and opening of that central channel of life force through the body, creating greater vitality.

Anuloma Viloma is alternate nostril breathing with no held breath retentions. It is very accessible and easy for most students to incorporate. I consider it a kriya or energy cleansing. *Nadi Shodhanam* pranayama is also an energy channel cleansing, yet it also uses the more subtle breath retentions which cultivate and direct prana on a more expansive level. For that reason, I cultivate *nadi shodhanam* as a pranayama. All of this is debatable, I am sure, so best not to get too caught up in the designations—the true potency comes in the practice.

PARTICULARS AND PRECAUTIONS

- Cultivates focus, balance, and relaxation.
- Appropriate any time of day/evening.
- Cultivate the 5:5 or 5:5:5:5 ratio; reduce if unsustainable, for example to 4:4 or 3:3.
- Avoid utilizing breath retentions when pregnant or suffering from acute asthma or lung issues.
- Full list of Immunity and Whole Health Benefits, page 218.

HOW TO DO ANULOMA VILOMA

Stabilize body, elongate spine, cultivating balance; sitting or reclined position can be used.

- Rest nondominant hand on the thigh in *Gyana Mudra* (thumb pad and index finger touching).
- With ring finger of dominant hand, close off the left nostril.

- Inhale through the right nostril for a slow 5-count, and then pause briefly at the top of the inhale to close both nostrils using ring finger and thumb of dominant hand.
- Exhale out the left nostril for 5 counts and pause briefly at the bottom of the exhalation. Stay on that side.
- Inhale through the left (same) nostril for a 5-count, pause briefly to close both nostrils, then switch.
- Exhale out the right nostril for 5 counts; pause briefly at the bottom of the exhalation. Stay on that side.
- Inhale through the right (same) nostril for a 5-count; pause briefly to close both nostrils, then switch.
- Continue in this pattern, creating box breathing within the alternating of the nostrils with no retentions.
- Repeat for three rounds: if sustainable and enjoyable, repeat for another eight rounds.
- Sit quietly for a minimum of one minute, observing how you feel, and to restore.
- Consider proceeding to one of the meditations shared in this book or to Shavasana/Corpse Pose.

HOW TO DO NADI SHODHANAM PRANAYAMA

Stabilize body, elongate spine, cultivating balance; sitting or reclined position can be used.

- Rest nondominant hand on the thigh in *Gyana Mudra* (thumb pad and index finger touching).
- With ring finger of dominant hand, close off the left nostril.
- Inhale through the right nostril for a slow 5-count, and then pause at the top of the inhale to retain the breath; close both nostrils using ring finger and thumb of dominant hand.
- Retain and hold the inhalation in for 5 counts, or equal to the length of inhalation.
- Exhale out the left nostril for 5 counts and pause at the bottom of the exhalation; stay on that side.

- Hold the breath out, retaining for 5 counts.
- Inhale through the left (same) nostril for a slow 5-count and then pause at the top of the inhale to retain the breath; close both nostrils.
- Retain and hold the inhalation in for 5 counts, or equal to the length of inhalation.
- Exhale out the right nostril for 5 counts and pause at the bottom of the exhalation; stay on that side.
- Hold the breath out, retaining for 5 counts.
- Inhale through the right (same) nostril for a slow 5 count and then pause at the top of the inhale to retain the breath, close both nostrils.
- Continue in this pattern, creating box breathing within the alternating of the nostrils.
- Repeat for three rounds. If sustainable and enjoyable, repeat for another eight rounds.
- Sit quietly for a minimum of one minute, observing how you feel, and to restore.
- Consider proceeding to one of the meditations shared in this book or to Shavasana/Corpse Pose.

TRATAKA KRIYA
(TRAH-TAH-KAH KREE-YA)
VISION CLEANSING

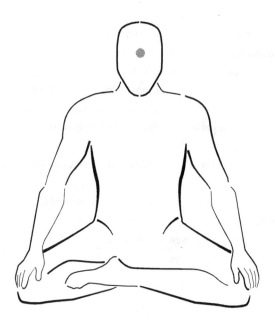

CONCENTRATION, CLARITY, OPENS INNER VISION, STRENGTHENS THE EYES

One of the Shat Kriyas or six essential cleansing tools described in the *Hatha Yoga Pradipika*, Trataka is a sustained relaxed gaze, pausing the blinking reflex and holding the eye's gaze on one point to clear the vision (it makes the eyes water and flushes them), strengthen the eye muscles, enhance concentration, and stimulate the pineal gland, which is associated with the third eye or inner vision. The practice cultivates focus, steadiness, and awareness. Various qualities can be cultivated by the choice of gazing point; for example, if mentally or physically overheated, gazing on water can cultivate a coolness and feeling of calm. When unfocused and scattered, gazing steadily at a flame can increase concentration and energy of clarity. As with all of these shared practices, trataka is to be practiced with gentleness, not straining or pushing, and cultivating compassion and a sense of balance. Trataka can be straining if overdone, limit to a one-minute maximum length of hold.

- Cultivates focus, balance, and relaxation.
- Appropriate any time of day/evening; recommended predawn/ after sunset.
- Limit to one-minute durations, maximum five-minute accumulative for an entire day.
- Stay upright for entire practice.
- Exercise caution when using a flame; take all appropriate fire hazard precautions.
- Avoid with glaucoma, epilepsy, schizophrenia, or tendencies toward hallucinations or eye issues.
- Full list of Immunity and Whole Health Benefits, page 218.

HOW TO DO IT

Stabilize body, elongate spine, cultivating balance; sitting posture is to be used.

- Breathe evenly through the nostrils; observe how you feel and create balance.
- Create *Gyana Mudra*/Wisdom Hand Seal in nondominant hand (see page 90), rest on thigh.
- Closing the dominant hand into a gentle fist, lift the thumb to be focal point.
- Align the thumb ten to twelve inches in front of your face.
- Relax the shoulders and entire body to cultivate steady/spacious.
- With a soft, relaxed gaze, suspend blinking and hold gaze on the thumb.
- Hold for up to one minute maximum, utilizing a slow and conscious 1:1 *sama vritti* breathing.
- Allow the eyes to water. Close the eyes when there is a sensation of burning or strain.

- Sit quietly for a minimum of one minute, observing how you feel, and to restore.
- Consider proceeding to one of the meditations shared in this book or to Shavasana/Corpse Pose.

TRATAKA DRISHTI OR GAZING POINTS

There are many *drishtis* or gazing points of attention for *trataka kriya*, for example, the *Shri Yantra* (sacred geometry of abundance) on the transition pages of this book, or an OM symbol, a candle flame, a dot, the full moon, a star, a rose, a body of water, a mirror, or anything that brings peace. I most often utilize my thumb, as it is very convenient and has an immediate centering effect on my system. Using the tip of the nose is also convenient, yet a little more challenging as a newer practitioner. Practice the nasal and third-eye gaze for ten-second holds with a maximum of no more than one minute, and then rest the eyes.

Any body of water can be used, even a glass of water, concentrating at the water line. Stay upright and in a calm alert state. The eyes will water, and you can continue to hold the gaze through the watering or close the eyes and bring the image into an inner vision hologram.

PRACTICES FOR FREEDOM

BRAHMARI PRANAYAMA
(BRAH-MAR-EE)
BEE BUZZING BREATH

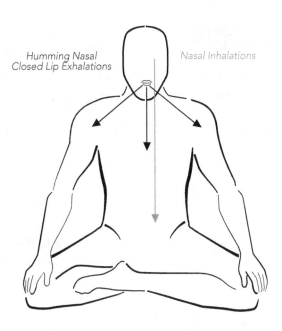

Humming Nasal
Closed Lip Exhalations

Nasal Inhalations

CLEARING, OPENING, EXPANDS CREATIVITY, ENHANCES
COGNITIVE FUNCTION

Creating a vibration, or buzzing, in the skull, sinuses, brain, throat, chest, and heart clears out stagnation and cultivates healing. In yoga traditions, *brahmari* is believed to bring the brain waves into gamma waves, which stimulate creativity, perception, and elevated states of consciousness. Studies have shown that ten minutes or more of practicing this vibrational breath boosts cognitive function as well as creating a nitric oxide super boost. Nitric oxide opens the blood vessels, increasing blood oxygen levels and reducing inflammation, and has been found to have a slew of whole health benefits for the entire body.

From a yogic perspective, this buzzing clears the head and draws awareness into the conscious heart and a place of quiet. Although most often practiced in a still seat, I have found this breathing to be effectively utilized in some basic asana, as well as in the shower or doing a quiet repetitive home task.

PARTICULARS AND PRECAUTIONS

- Increases the production of nitric oxide, aiding in oxygen circulation.
- Stimulates the throat, thyroid gland, vocal cords, tongue, sinuses, and pineal gland.
- Pushes stale air particles out of the deeper areas of the lungs, throat, and mouth.
- Appropriate for morning to late afternoon; avoid before bedtime.
- Can be utilized with various mudras and facial pressure points.
- Avoid pushing for volume on vocal cords, and only practice as feels sustainable.
- Avoid breath practice if experiencing instability or lightheadedness.
- Avoid if neck, throat, sinus, or nasal injury, or acute high or low blood pressure, history of stroke, diagnosed schizophrenia, or acute trauma.
- Full list of Immunity and Whole Health Benefits, page 218.

HOW TO DO IT

Stabilize body, elongate spine, cultivating balance; sitting or reclined position can be used.

- Exhale the breath completely out and pause it for a moment.
- Breathe evenly through the nostrils; observe how you feel and create balance.
- Inhale through the nostrils with a gentle pulling or soft snoring sound.
- Exhale with the mouth closed, to create a high-pitched buzzing like the vibration of a bee.

- Repeat three times and then add gentle pressure to the inner cartilage of the ears.
- With tips of the index fingers, gently press to close the entrance of the ears by pressing on the cartilage.
- Cultivate the breath ratio 5:5 or 6:6 for three rounds.
- Release the fingers from the ears, palms down, breathing naturally, feeling the effects of the practice.
- Sit quietly for a minimum of one minute, observing how you feel and to restore.
- Consider proceeding to one of the meditations shared in this book or to Shavasana/Corpse Pose.

Another simplified and tactile version is utilizing the humming with ZZZZ and SHZZZ sounds. Use the hands either to cup the ears or as a gentle vibration baffle in front of the nose, sinuses, and throat. Inhale through both nostrils as you exhale one round of ZZZZ humming vibration through nose and lips, and then the following round with the exhalation of SHZZZZ. Alternate back and forth to create a strong vibration through the chest, throat, and skull. I find this version very accessible to many as an introduction to the above practice, as well as very helpful when teaching, in speaking with clarity and distinction.

GARDABHA-SIMHA-BHUJANGA-BIDALA KRIYA

DONKEY, LION, SNAKE, AND CAT CLEANSING

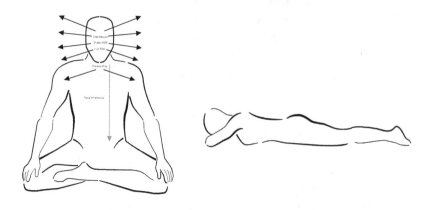

WARMING, CLEARING, TENSION AND EMOTION RELEASING

A donkey, a lion, a snake, and a cat walk into a bar...and they share a shot of the nitric oxide boost. Here we move right into the toning vibration of throat-clearing donkey, then into the roar of the lion, the hiss of the snake, and the meow of the cat. Creating a stable of clearing and stimulating vibrations, aiding in circulation and inducing the rest/digest response as well as releasing held emotional tension out of the system. Each of these vibrations have roots in passed on yogic *kriyas*. I have experienced that the donkey clears stubborn frustration, the lion activates courage to face truth, the snake purges the venom of anger, and the cat meows to reconnect and open the pathway to love and inner vision. These can be practiced on the belly or in an upright seat.

PARTICULARS AND PRECAUTIONS

- Releases facial and mental/emotional tension into relaxation.
- Stimulates the abdominal cavity, throat, thyroid gland, vocal cords, tongue, and sinuses.

- Pushes stale air particles out of the deeper areas of the lungs, throat, mouth, and sinuses.
- Appropriate for morning to late afternoon; avoid before bedtime.
- Avoid pushing for volume on vocal cords, and only practice as feels sustainable.
- Avoid breath practice if experiencing instability or lightheadedness.
- Avoid if neck or throat injury, history of high blood pressure, heart problems, epilepsy, hernia, or recent abdominal surgery, or if pregnant.

HOW TO DO DONKEY (NOSE INHALE, LIPS CLOSED, "HAY" OR GLOTTAL INHALATION) AND LION (EXHALE MOUTH "HAAH")

Stabilize body, elongate spine, cultivating balance; sitting or prone belly reclined position can be used.

- Breathe evenly through the nostrils; observe how you feel and create balance.
- Inhale through the nostrils while gently closing the throat, similar to Ujjayi breathing, making the beginning sound of a donkey-like bray (not too strong! Just enough for a gentle massage).
- Exhale, pushing tongue behind bottom teeth, or with tongue stretched out to chin, creating Lion's Breath clearing.
- Repeat slowly a minimum of three times, up to a maximum of eight.
- Proceed to Snake hissing.

HOW TO DO SNAKE (INHALE NOSE/EXHALE MOUTH "HISSSS")

- Inhale through the nostrils.
- Exhale, creating a steady snake hissing sound out the mouth, pushing out the "venom" of anger or frustration that may be in the body through the emphasized SSS.
- Repeat slowly a minimum of three times, up to a maximum of eight.
- Proceed to Cat meowing.

- Inhale through the nostrils.
- Exhale with the lips closed, steadily making the ME sound up behind the nose, inside the head in a high-pitched MEEEOW repetition. Extend and emphasize the EEE portion of the meow.
- Repeat slowly a minimum of three times, up to a maximum of eight.
- Feel free to explore octaves and tempo changes to create release and joy.
- Afterward, if on belly, turn ear to one side, or sit quietly, breathing evenly through the nostrils. Observe the effects of the practice.
- Consider proceeding to *Hasya Kriya*/Ha-ha Cleansing or Shavasana/ Corpse Pose.

HASYA KRIYA
(HAHS-YA KREE-YA)
HA-HA CLEANSING

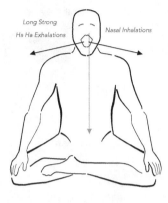

Long Strong
Ha Ha Exhalations

Nasal Inhalations

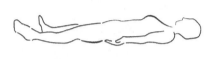

CLEARING, JOY, RELAXATION, RELEASE OF "HAPPY" HORMONES

Laughter is indeed the best medicine and, in my experience, this Ha-ha can easily shift back and forth between tears and laughter. Both are wonderful relievers of stress and health boosters.

Try the Ha-ha out first, and then close the lips and take the practice more inward. Sit or recline quietly in stillness afterwards to integrate and feel the effects.

PARTICULARS AND PRECAUTIONS

- Stimulates the happy hormones of dopamine, serotonin, oxytocin, and endorphins.
- Stimulates the abdominal cavity, throat, thyroid gland, vocal cords, tongue, and sinuses.
- Pushes stale air particles out of the deeper areas of the lungs, throat, and mouth.
- Appropriate for morning to late afternoon; avoid before bedtime.

- Avoid pushing for volume on vocal cords, and only practice as feels sustainable.
- Avoid breath practice if experiencing instability or lightheadedness.
- Avoid if neck or throat injury, history of high blood pressure, heart problems, epilepsy, hernia, or recent abdominal surgery, or if pregnant.

HOW TO DO IT

Stabilize body, elongate spine, cultivating balance; sitting or reclined position can be used.

- Breathe evenly through the nostrils; observe how you feel and create balance.
- Inhale through the nostrils a full and satisfying breath.
- Exhale out the mouth with a sturdy HA-HA, continue Ha-ha-ha, slowly building a sustainable speed until you naturally laugh, cry, or are comfortably fatigued.
- Reset in stillness with a quiet, natural breath to stabilize.
- Consider repeating, and if it feels easily accessible, create the inner laughter with lips closed.
- Grow from a slow to a sustainable faster speed until you naturally laugh, cry, or are comfortably fatigued.
- Stabilize in stillness with a quiet, natural breath; recline in Shavasana/ Corpse Pose to observe the effects.

PRACTICES FOR WHOLE-BEING INTEGRATION

SHUSHUMNA KRIYA
(SHU-SHOOM-NAH KREE-YA)
JOYFUL MIND (UNISON NOSTRIL) BREATHING

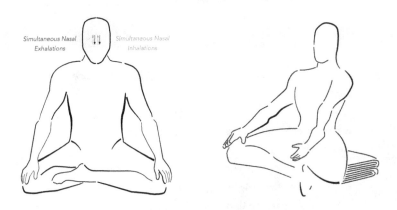

Simultaneous Nasal Exhalations

Simultaneous Nasal Inhalations

JOY, FOCUS, BALANCE, INTEGRATION

The shifting of nostril dominance is a normal and natural occurrence throughout the day. When we alternate the nostril dominance, as in the previous practices *anuloma viloma* and *nadi shodhanam*, we gently balance the mind and calm the system in preparation for the movement of joyful healing energy through the entire system. The opened channel of balanced, joyful *pranic* energy is called *shushumna nadi*. This simple breathing technique is to be practiced after three or so rounds of alternate nostril breathing and involves shifting into simultaneous nostril breathing to open that central channel. Syncing up the movement of the breath and life force up and down the energetic channels, bringing balance to the physical hemispheres of the brain, into the subtle balance of the energy polarities of "ha tha" or Sun/Moon, called *ida* and *pingala*. This opens a central channel of awareness and vitality, creating an experience of unity of mind, body and spirit, or yoga.

- Stimulates the frontal lobe of the brain and the pineal gland.
- Cultivates joy, vitality, clarity, focus, balance, and integration.
- Appropriate any time of day/evening; excellent just prior to sleep.
- Can be practiced in conjunction with Ujjayi and Box Breathing.
- Cultivate steady and spacious within effort and body; avoid any strain or over-ambition.
- Full Rest/Digest Benefits, page 66.

HOW TO DO IT

Stabilize body, elongate spine, cultivating balance; sitting or reclined position can be used.

- Breathe evenly through the nostrils; observe how you feel and create balance.
- Create *Gyana Mudra/*Wisdom Hand Seal in both hands (see page 90).
- Exhale the breath slowly through both of the nostrils in unison.
- Inhale slowly in unison through both nostrils, tracing the air from the nasal flares to the eyebrow center.
- Cultivate a *sama vritti*, a balanced ratio, within the unison nostril breath.
- Observe the quality as you move to breathing more slowly and fully with each round of breath.
- Continue for eight rounds, or as long as it feels nourishing.

SAMI KARANA PRANAYAMA

CHANNELS COMING TOGETHER MEDITATION

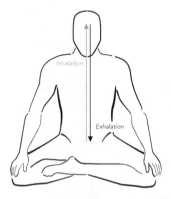
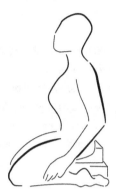

BALANCE OF POLARITIES, INTEGRATION, EXPANDED CONSCIOUSNESS

As someone who enjoys eating *and cooking* and is of Italian-American descent, my go-to ingredients for many meals are good-quality olive oil and raw garlic. It is always delicious, effective, and super versatile. The same goes as a yogi with this foundational energy-balancing meditation. This meditation is the *aglio e olio* (olive oil and garlic) of yoga energy meditations (at least in my viewpoint, *che bello!).*

This balancing breathing meditation can stand alone or be adapted into other more intricate explorations. It will do the job of calming the mind, balancing the entire system, and opening up the central channel, *shushumna nadi*, of vitality and joy. Integrate this one into your regular practice and you will have the basis of great healing for your entire life journey.

PARTICULARS AND PRECAUTIONS

- Stimulates the frontal lobe of the brain and the pineal gland.
- Cultivates joy, vitality, clarity, focus, balance, and integration.
- Appropriate any time of day/evening; excellent just prior to sleep.
- Full Rest/Digest Benefits, page 66.

Stabilize body, elongate spine, cultivating balance; sitting or reclined position can be used.

- Breathe evenly through the nostrils; observe how you feel and create balance.
- Close the eyes and bring inner awareness to the base of the spine.
- Create *Gyana Mudra/*Wisdom Hand Seal in both hands (see page 90).
- With your inner vision, slowly inhale to trace a warm golden light on the breath from the base of the spine, through the navel, the chest, the throat, and the middle of the eyebrows, up to the crown of the head.
- On the exhalation, trace a cool blue light on the breath slowly back down the midline to the base.
- Continue to cultivate the warm solar yellow on ascending inhalation and cool lunar blue on descending exhalation to balance polarities and open the central channel of energy in the system.
- Cultivate a balanced, slow, satisfying, and sustainable breath pattern.
- Remain breathing, sitting quietly, effortlessly following the breath, until completely quiet in absorption.
- Consider reclining in Shavasana/Corpse Pose when the body is ready to restore and reset.

AROHANA AVAROHANA
(AHR-OH-WAHN-AH UH-WAHR-UH-HAHN-AH)
INFINITY MEDITATION

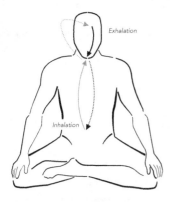

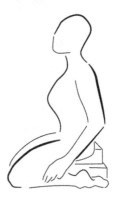

CALMING, BALANCES POLARITIES, INTEGRATION, EXPANDS CONSCIOUSNESS

As the final practice for our exploration, I offer a more intricate, potent, and a personal favorite of concentration practices. I first learned this figure-eight infinity meditation practice from one of my most influential yoga teachers, Alan Finger, and I believe it originally comes from the teachings of Yogananda Paramahamsa, who was one of Alan's' father Mani Finger's primary yoga teachers. It brings the energy of consciousness through the chakra system, opening up psychic pathways. You may notice that the foundational movement of this meditation is similar to the foundational Sami Karana, Channels Coming Together Meditation. By nature, the Arohana, the ascending inhalation, opens us up and the Avarohana, the descending back passage, guides us to surrender or integration. I tend to utilize this practice when I am looking to unblock creativity, open up a sense of possibility, and connect to cosmic support.

PARTICULARS AND PRECAUTIONS

- Stimulates the frontal lobe of the brain and the pineal gland.
- Cultivates joy, vitality, clarity, focus, balance, and integration.
- Balances *pranic* passageways and cultivates expanded consciousness.

- Appropriate any time of day/evening.
- Full Rest/Digest Benefits, page 66.

Stabilize body, elongate spine, cultivating balance; sitting or reclined position can be used.

- Breathe evenly through the nostrils; observe how you feel and create balance.
- Close the eyes and bring inner awareness to the base of the spine.
- Create *Gyana Mudra*/Wisdom Hand Seal in both hands (see page 90).
- With your inner vision, slowly inhale to trace a golden light on the breath from the base of the spine, through the navel, the chest, entering into the jugular notch at the throat, continuing to the back of the head, up over the crown into the midbrain just behind the eyebrow center.
- On the exhalation, the light shifts to blue and moves out through the eyebrow center, descending down through the throat into C7, the bottom back of the neck, down the back body to the base of the spine.
- Gently lift the chin as the inhalation moves through the sacral, solar plexus, and heart areas before deepening into the throat notch, and then gently lower the chin just lower than parallel to the floor as the consciousness moves to the tuft area at the back of the head, up and over to the space of the fontanelle at the top of the head, before landing near the pineal gland at midbrain.
- The exhalation slides down into the front of the throat into the back of the neck, descending and releasing through the back of the heart, posterior solar plexus, and sacral area, returning to the base.
- Cultivate a balanced, slow, satisfying, and sustainable breath pattern.
- Once fully stabilized, explore a gentle retention at the top of the inhalation to open up inner vision.
- Remain breathing, sitting quietly, effortlessly following the breath, until completely quiet in absorption.
- Consider reclining in Shavasana/Corpse Pose when the body is ready to restore and reset.

CHAPTER 12

SEQUENCES FOR INTEGRATION

Although this is our last chapter of sequences, this is truly just a jumping-off point. The following sequences in this chapter are simply some good, nourishing entry points for you to integrate the many tools in this book and beyond as your yoga journey develops.

These are a sampling of different types of practices, including mild illness support, gentle illness recovery, basic restorative, multiple levels of strength and vitality practices, which are longer in length so a bit more complex, and a well-rounded balanced pranayama sequence.

Whenever you come to a pose that has two sides, such as Lunge Pose, automatically know to do both sides, and of course always do both sides with equal quality and duration.

Again, these are just an introduction to the many amazing meals that can be created with the tools in this book. Collaborate with me and once more familiar with stringing poses together, begin to make your own.

The following sequences are in this order

1.   Balancing Pranayama/Meditation Integrated Sequence
2.   Basic Restorative Integrated Sequence
3.   Mild Illness Support Integrated Sequence
4.   Gentle Illness Recovery Integrated Sequence
5.   Gentle Balanced Integrated Sequence
6.   Basic Strength Vitality Integrated Sequence

#1
BALANCING PRANAYAMA/MEDITATION
INTEGRATED SEQUENCE

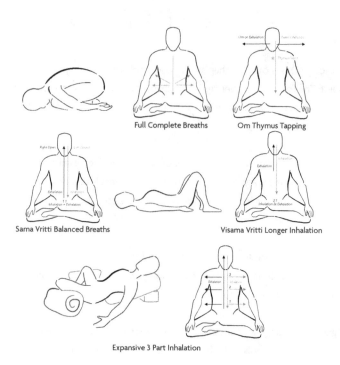

Full Complete Breaths

Om Thymus Tapping

Sama Vritti Balanced Breaths

Visama Vritti Longer Inhalation

Expansive 3 Part Inhalation

Transition through fetal position

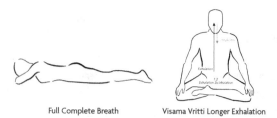

Full Complete Breath

Visama Vritti Longer Exhalation

Transition through fetal position on Right Side

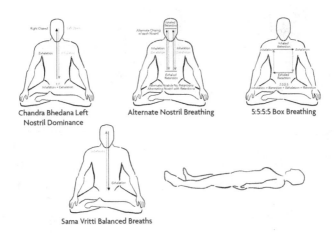

Chandra Bhedana Left
Nostril Dominance

Alternate Nostril Breathing

5:5:5:5 Box Breathing

Sama Vritti Balanced Breaths

#2
BASIC RESTORATIVE INTEGRATED SEQUENCE

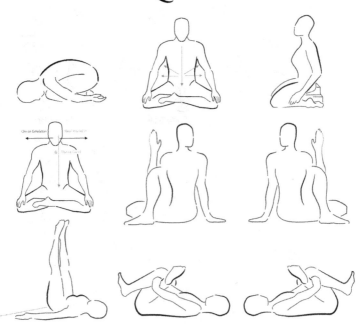

Transition through fetal position

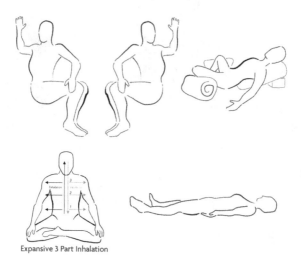

Expansive 3 Part Inhalation

#3
MILD ILLNESS SUPPORT INTEGRATED SEQUENCE

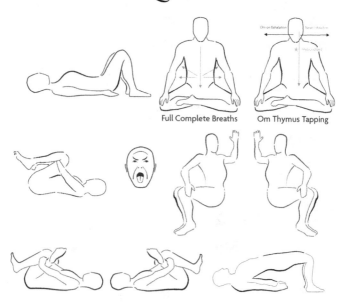

Full Complete Breaths   Om Thymus Tapping

Transition through fetal position, move onto belly

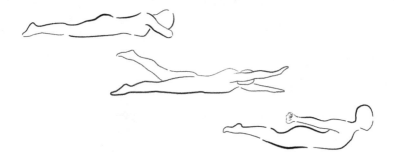

Transition through fetal position, return to back

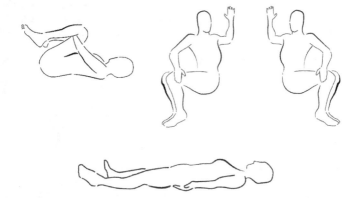

#4
GENTLE ILLNESS RECOVERY INTEGRATED SEQUENCE

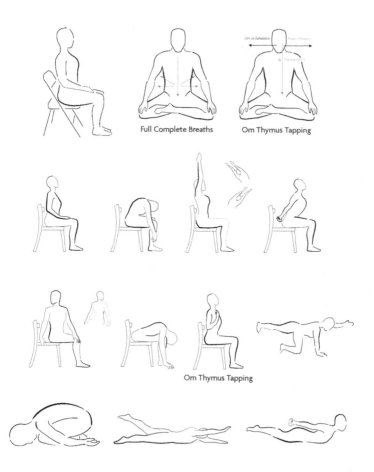

Full Complete Breaths

Om Thymus Tapping

Om Thymus Tapping

Transition through fetal position

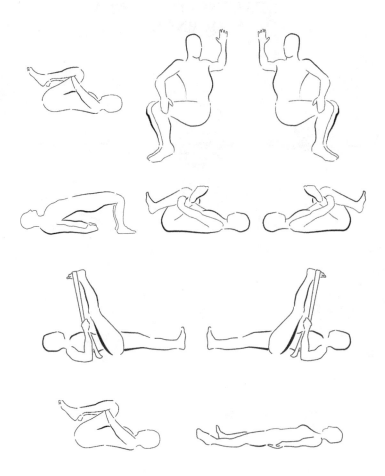

#5
GENTLE BALANCED INTEGRATED SEQUENCE

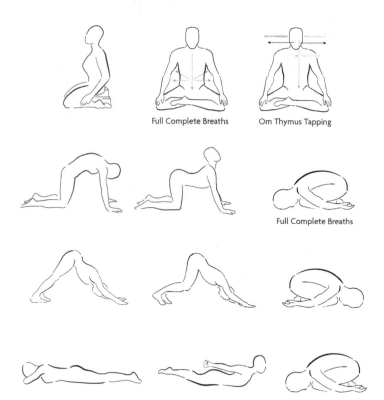

Full Complete Breaths

Om Thymus Tapping

Full Complete Breaths

Transition to standing

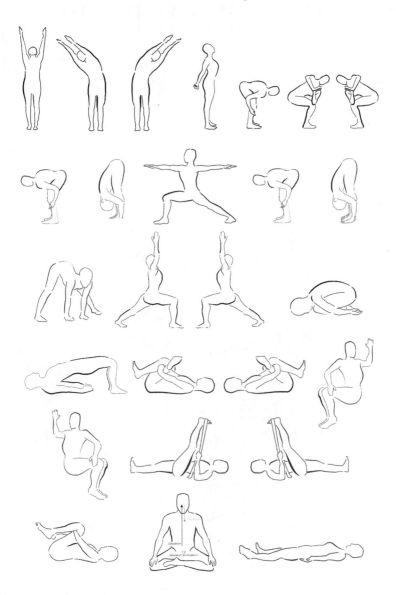

#6
STRENGTH VITALITY INTEGRATED SEQUENCE

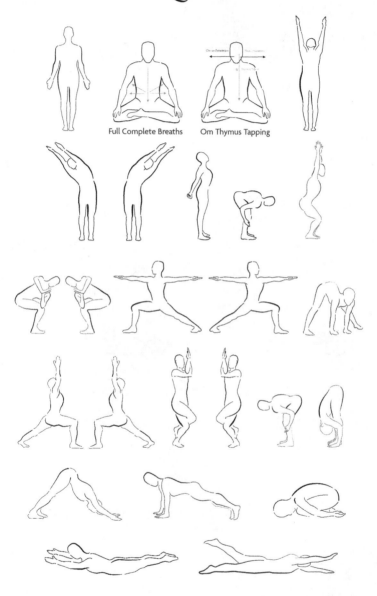

Full Complete Breaths   Om Thymus Tapping

Transition through fetal position

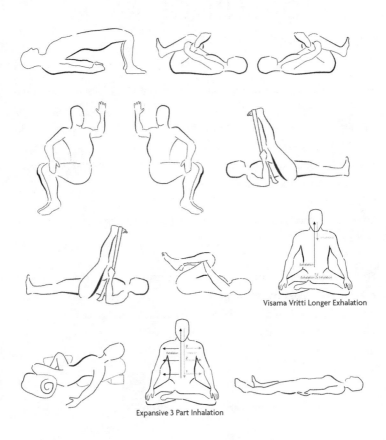

Visama Vritti Longer Exhalation

Expansive 3 Part Inhalation

CHAPTER 13

OPENINGS AND CLOSINGS

How you begin and end has importance. An integrated yoga practice has shifted and healed almost every aspect of my life. Over the years, it has transformed my mind, my body, and my relationships. Through this study and practice I have slowly and steadily created my life to be my practice. It is how I wake up in the morning, prepare myself for the day, take care of my home and family, and navigate my work, and how I close each and every day.

One thing I often hear from students and friends is, "Life is so busy, how do you do it?"

From this question, I conclude our yogic exploration here by sharing some of my lifestyle integrations. My hope is to give real-life inspiration on what a daily healing yoga practice can look like and how you can be motivated to create your own, just-right-for-you yoga healing practice.

This is what it looks like for *me*.

Mom of three, full-time teacher and regular person.

This is how I generally do it.

First, I focus on the openings, the closings, and the transitions for my most mindful attention. Whether it is the mundane every day or the more expansive openings and closings that align with lunar cycles, seasonal cycles, and life events, I put my attention there first.

For my every day, I have set practices that are habits in place at the beginning and end of the day, that stabilize and focus me and create a long-term accumulative effect of whole health.

OPENINGS, CLOSINGS, AND TRANSITIONS

Focus on building habits and helpful systems around the opening of the day or event, the closing, and any key transitions. An example of key transitions is the practice of pausing, breathing, and connecting with a deeper intention before choosing with which foot to step through a doorway. Once practiced, this can be an effective and efficient moment of plugging into the energy of healing and mindfulness throughout the day.

Here is my average day, in its possibly boring and mundane steps, I hope it is helpful!

A.M.

I most often wake naturally before dawn. I wasn't always an early riser, yet in these years I find that the wee hours just before dawn are precious, sacred, and feel essential for my well-being, so knowing that, my body wakes me up early most days. I usually shift my position to turn supine on my back, stretch out to create symmetry and balance in my body. I practice conscious breathing through my nose (sama vritti, Full Complete Breaths) and feel through my body for sensations and information of imbalance. I personally practice prayer, and at this time I usually connect with an inner prayer of gratitude for waking up, for my life, for the earth, and for my loved ones. I also usually inquire, "What is important for me right now? What am I to pay attention to today?" If I am feeling a lack of clarity, I will make a request: "Guide me, show me the way of love today." Then I feel and listen to what comes into my awareness. I usually close my prayer with a request for unconditional love and compassion to heal every cell of my body and to support all who come in contact with me. I imagine that love and light warming and radiating within me before I move on.

I open my eyes and most often take time to see the last of the stars in the night sky or the faint glow of dawn. I practice some deeper breathing, such as Three-Part Expansive Breaths. I begin to imagine my day, mentally walking through the sequence of the day, doing an inner rehearsal of anything that feels like it could use more intention and energetic support. If there is something I am challenged by or unsure of, I will walk through the steps, imagining and experiencing success, before I get out of bed.

I take my time getting out of bed. I go slow, roll to my side, and take my feet over the side to pause seated before I proceed. I create a brief proper seat, anchoring my feet, elongating my spine, again taking an inventory, balancing my breath, and connecting into my intention for the day. I stand up slowly, as usually my body is very stiff from the inactivity, and I feel through my body. I create Mountain Pose and anchor my feet to rise tall. Again I breathe and, like a flash of lightning, connect into my intention.

I use the bathroom where I pause to breathe, briefly stretch my body, and connect to my vison and intention again while washing my hands and walking out the door. As mentioned, my practice is to pay extra attention to transitions, especially when I walk through doorways. I try to mindfully walk through connecting to the present moment and breathing into whatever is important. Honestly, I don't remember to focus on every single doorway, yet when I do remember, it is immediately aligning and helpful.

I always go right into the kitchen from the bathroom in the morning. It is one of those dependable habits that I build on, and for that reason I do the bulk of my morning healing practices at this time.

Some people have a kitchen junk drawer; I have a kitchen self-care drawer, and that is where I go first, as it has all my tools for my yogic *dinecharya* (DEEN-a-CHAR-ee-ah) or first morning cleansing routine.

In the dark of early morning, right at the kitchen sink, while my whole house sleeps, I begin my cleansing routine. I scrape my tongue with my copper tongue scraper to clear impurities that my body has detoxed. I floss and brush my teeth. I use the water I set out on the counter overnight, that is now room temperature, to take my thyroid pill to support my healing from Hashimoto hypothyroidism. I drink about sixteen ounces at that time. I then clear my nose and sinuses by using sterile saline wash with a copper *neti* pot. (I have that boiled, prepped from the night before, water at room temperature in a clean jar, ready to go.) I do a brief series of *Kapalabhati* breaths after *neti* to clear my nose and head of excess water and warm myself up.

I then stimulate and exfoliate my skin by gently dry-brushing my face, neck, and whatever skin is exposed with a small, clean, natural-bristle skin brush. Then I briefly steam and wash my face. I add a mixture of rose hip oil and aloe as a moisturizer to my skin, face, hands, and feet with a little massage. I use coconut oil to oil pull my teeth and gums while I am care taking my face and skin.

While swishing to clean my gums, I also prep my meditation seat, my favorite blanket, my journal, and whatever book I am studying (I am foremost a student and I find it important to continue studying each day). If it is a writing day, I also place my laptop and notes just to the side of my meditation cushion. I spit the oil in the garbage (never the sink). I clear my mouth with fresh water. I say a quick prayer of thanks and a flash of intention for the next step. I stretch my spine in all directions with a Sun Stretch Series, including spinal rotation with a couple of detox poses; then I take my meditation seat.

This morning sequence took a fair amount of study, prep, and trial and error to come to. I planned it out, and every day I set up what is needed the night before. Because of the preparation, as well as the repetition of doing it many times, it only takes me about twenty minutes from beginning to end. This morning sequence boosts my immune system and whole health in all the ways that we have explored in this book, and even a few more! In my view, it is a key bundle of habits that supports my vitality and gets my whole system aligned.

For my breathing and meditation practice, I usually sit in a lifted cross-legged or kneeling seat, and I always start my practice with a series of morning Sanskrit peace mantras that have been passed on to me over the years by my teachers. They calm and focus me into a stillness. I do a series of pranayamas based on how

I feel, my energy level, the season, and what is needed. I practice a simple focused awareness meditation and sit quietly in stillness for from as little as ten minutes to as long as fifty minutes, depending on the day. I sit for a shorter time when I have a writing deadline (like today!), or if it is a school day and the kids need help with breakfast. I will have a longer practice on a more spacious weekend morning. After practice, I write, self-study journal, read/study, practice more asana, ride my spin bike, or make gluten free French toast for my husband and kids (my favorite, yum).

After my practice, before breakfast, on an empty stomach, I drink another sixteen ounces of clean water, this time with juice from a half of lemon or lime, ionized zinc, and a probiotic mineral supplement. After fifteen minutes, I drink sixteen ounces of freshly-juiced organic celery juice, which helps detox my digestive tract and helps me with the symptoms and healing journey with the aforementioned autoimmune issues. Over the past decade, I went from debilitating symptoms, including quarter-size hives all over my body every day, to being mostly symptom-free, and (hallelujah!) no hives. This is one of the inspirations for me to share these practices with you and write this book.

I connect with and hug all my people, and I help them get going on their day of work and school meetings. Then I make coffee. Yes, I do. I add supplements, including healing mushroom powders, into my coffee. This helps me believe this coffee practice is helpful to my whole health. (Debatable, I know!) I did say that I am a *regular* person, right?

I usually wait to eat my first meal fourteen hours or so after my last meal to help rest my digestion. I practice making the food for myself and family with intentions of love and gratitude. Sometimes, I have to admit, there is a lot of chaos and pressure happening in the kitchen, yet often enough I am able to come back to blessing our food with love and intention before we eat it. It is a work in progress.

During the morning, I help my first-grader with his schoolwork (we are in remote schooling) while I also sit doing administration tasks like emails and updates for projects and teaching. Late morning, I will go into my yoga studio and lead practices on a livestream. I will stay in the studio after and do some specific poses to help my body for the day (although I physically do the poses with many of my classes, this is important so I can tune in to my own body's needs). I say mantras of peaceful intentions as I enter/open my studio and as I close it after sessions.

P.M.

I drink more clean water. I help my family with lunch, although often they are on their own with this meal. I have lunch and connect, and then rest a bit after, sometimes sitting outside in the air or sun if the weather permits or taking a twenty-minute Shavasana. Later, I will walk on the grass, dirt and land around my home and breathe. I prep dinner, I take care of our family animals, and I clean or tidy the house. I utilize all of this time for practicing intentions and adding in postures and breathing whenever natural. I practice staying mindful of my energy and the cues my body and emotions are giving me. I may study more or do an hour of writing or work before the end of the day.

Toward later afternoon and early evening, we all come together as a whole family and connect, talk, and play something either outside for a more active game or play, or inside for a rousing board game—our favorite is Sorry!. That game never gets old and always creates a lot of laughter. I see this connection and play time as being as important as my postures and routines; it is part of my healing practice.

I drink more clean water. I finish making dinner sometimes with a glass of red wine, oftentimes with music on, singing and dancing while cooking in my kitchen. We sit down to eat dinner. We most always, if possible, sit together for dinner. We start dinner with each person sharing a couple of things they are grateful for at the beginning of the meal, before we dig in. We try to make meals relaxed and happy. We usually all clean up after dinner—well, maybe not all, as the littlest guy is usually running around us playing. Then, maybe another board game or, one of my favorites, we watch a Warriors basketball game. Go Warriors! Then I begin to prep myself and my kids for bed. I try to wean them off devices by dinnertime or soon after. Some days are better than others; getting off tech is again a work in progress.

I prepare my tools for my morning cleansing routine and practices for the morning. I set up and organize all that I can. I write down my to-do list, which includes the steps of my routines and practices and put the paper out where I can see it first thing. I put out any special supplements or things I need to remember for the next day. I help my kids do the same for their next day.

BEDTIME

I close my day with a shorter nighttime cleansing sequence. I bathe or shower, wash my face. I floss and brush. I massage some nourishing lotion onto my face, hands, and feet. I hug all my people and tell them I love them. Then I get into bed, usually around nine thirty.

I do the reverse of my morning breathing and reset. I stretch out on my back and create symmetry in my body. I usually cover my eyes with a lightly weighted eye pillow and slow down my breath. I usually practice uneven exhalation breath and quiet myself down. I say a prayer of gratitude. I imagine my loved ones, one at a time, happy, healthy, and safe. I feel myself happy, healthy, and safe. Then I fall asleep. Sleep is a priority for me and, as I wake early, I try to get to bed early enough for a minimum of seven to eight hours of sleep.

That is a view into my whole-day yoga practice. It is steeped in repetition and habits of self-study and listening to my inner cues, redirecting my mind to positive possibility and mindful intentions, consciously breathing, and moving my body in ways to support its health and balance. This is my yoga, and you will have *your* yoga. It may have moments of similarity, yet it will be uniquely yours.

Cultivate another step deeper into *your yoga* by creating a mini morning or evening cleansing routine that you use in conjunction with breathing and mindfulness to support your body's detox and your nervous system reset to healing.

We can inspire each other to keep going and *oh well* to what feels like failure or challenge. We can learn from each other and help teach each other. It's circular, not linear, and it is a perfectly imperfect practice.

I hope this more personal view is helpful and that there are some good breadcrumbs as well as juicy meals in this book that nourish you and help guide you along your path to fullness, vitality, strong immunity, and radiant whole health.

I would love to hear from you and how your practice is going. Don't hesitate to reach out. Just go to my site at www.melaniesalvatoreaugust.com and send me a note. I'm on Facebook and Instagram too, so if that is your thing, we can connect there as well. There are also lots of helpful resources on my site and additional study opportunities to support your journey with and beyond this book. Check them out, surround yourself with support, and lovingly, gently, in a *feel-good* way, keep going!

Thank you for going on this healing journey with me.

> May we together be supported.
> May we together feel safe to be vulnerable and earnest students of yoga (and life).
> May we together be transformed by that vulnerability and earnestness. Let that be the energy of our transformation and healing.
> As all things are impermanent except for peace, when we part, may we part in peace.
> And may all who come in contact with us be touched by that peace.

—A personal translation of the peace and collaboration mantra from the *Upanishads: Saha Nau Avantuu.*

Sending out love and peace to you,

"ONLY ONE THING? DO THIS."

Chapter 9

Focus on what is *easy to integrate* and *feels good* as the foundation to build your daily practice on.

Chapter 10

Make Shavasana/Corpse Pose a priority (consider joining me in the Twenty-One-Day Shavasana/Corpse Pose Practice Inspiration), practice five to twenty minutes daily with gentle deep breaths through the nose.

Chapter 11

Practice Unison Nostril Breaths, page 237, before rising out of bed and falling asleep each night as a potent "hack."

Chapter 12/13

Create a cleansing morning or nighttime routine, whichever feels easiest to begin. Focus attention on openings, closings, and simple transitions to further develop your practice.

RESOURCES

These are just a few...there are many many more!

Bhagavad Gita by Eknath Easwaran

Yoga Sutras of Patanjali by Sri Swami Satchidananda

The Secret of the Yoga Sutras by Pandit Rajmani Tigunait

Light on Pranayama by BKS Iyengar

Heart of Yoga by TKV Desikachar

The Yoga of Breath: A Step-by-Step Guide to Pranayama by Richard Rosen

Yoga—Ancient Heritage, Tomorrow's Vision by Indu Arora

Mudras—The Sacred Secret by Indu Arora

Ayurveda and Marma Therapy by David Frawley

Restore and Rebalance; Restful Yoga for Stressful Times by Judith Hanson Lasater

Yoga Mind, Body, Spirit by Donna Farhi

Eastern Body, Western Mind by Anodea Judith

Chakra Yoga by Alan Finger

Metahuman by Deepak Chopra

Deep Listening by Jillian Pransky

Breath by James Nestor

Living Yoga: 52 Weeks of Inspiration to Center and Enhance Everyday Life by Rachel Scott

Becoming Supernatural by Joe Dispenza

The Surrender Experiment by Michael A. Singer

The Humming Effect by Jonathan Goldman

Essentialism: The Disciplined Pursuit of Less by Greg McKeown

Atomic Habits by James Clear

The Habit Trip by Sarah Hays Coomer

The Seat of the Soul by Gary Zukav

The Path Made Clear by Oprah Winfrey

My favorite yoga props

Manduka (mat, blocks)
Chattra (bolsters, cushions)

My favorite streaming yoga service (catch me here!)

athome.yogaworks.com
JustBeYoga.com

ACKNOWLEDGMENTS

I am deeply grateful for the gifts that have been given to me over the years to study and learn about the healing arts. Starting way back in the eighties, when the local mall had an actual bookstore with a section on yoga and self-help. *Creative Visualization* by Shakti Gawain blew my young mind and guided me on this path of seeking and wholeness.

Thank you to Oprah Winfrey, who gave me one of my earliest exposures to so many thought leaders. How I loved coming home from school to watch your show. You are such an elite teacher, and I am forever grateful for the courage and fortitude it must have taken to forge the path that you have for so many of us.

For the study of the human condition at the University of North Carolina School for the Arts, what an amazing playground to see, feel, and do, versus simply theorize. Special love to my masterful teachers who helped me open: Robert Francesconi, Martin Rader, Felix Ivanov, Yury and Tanya Belov, Cigdem Onat, and Robert Moyer.

To the thoughtful, kind, earnest, dedicated and generous yoga teachers who have helped me find my way as a student and a teacher over the last twenty-five years, from NYC, LA, and Northern California, thank you.

To the many behind-the-scenes angels who have supported and guided me through the amazing learning ground that is YogaWorks as well as ISHTA Yoga. Behind those sparkling studio spaces and that global reach is a heartbeat of true kindness and authentic yoga. So much of my integrated practices come from you. Years ago, when you guided me on the teacher trainer path, I hit the lottery. As I look back, the growth is mind-blowing. I am forever grateful for all the education and opportunity in this journey.

Big thanks to my early readers who suffered through terrible organization and punctuation; love you Mary Foriero Patel, Marissa and Jamie Muth, Dr Ali Sadrieh, and Sanskrit Jon (Jon Janaka).

Special thanks to Alan Finger, Elena Brower, Mark Whitwell, Mynx Inatsugu, Jon Janaka, Rachel Scott, and Indu Arora, who have personally blessed me with life-changing teachings and showed me authentic examples of living your yoga.

To the radiant, humble, brilliant, and kind sister from afar, Sarah Platt Finger. Thank you for the many years of kindnesses and inspiration. Thank you for writing such a beautiful and thoughtful foreword; your generosity is humbling. I am so glad you are in this wild world.

To the Mango Publishing and Yellow Pear Press teams, wow, you are all so top-notch. You are as kind as you are brilliant. Thank you for believing in me and supporting me in bringing these healing and life-changing practices to many more friends. Heartfelt thank you to Robin Miller, such a kind human and masterful copy editor as well as the wonderful Morgane Leoni whose amazing design took complex material and made it truly accessible. You are both so deeply appreciated.

To Amanda Alappat, who volunteered her most talented and brilliant husband, Sebastian Alappat, to create the artwork for this book, such gratitude! You two are elite and gorgeous from the inside out. To Sebastian Alappat, you are like my long-lost spirit brother; thank you for all your talent, grace, and patience as we worked out the beautiful flow of this artwork. You are a bright star.

To the life-changer, the woman with an amazing heart, fantastic eye, and impeccable intuition, Lisa Duncan McGuinness, writer, publisher, editor, and talent-developer extraordinaire. Our now-long-running collaboration story is one of pure spirit, delight, and exceptional timings. Thank you for believing in me and mentoring me so gently in this cool book world all along the way. You embody fierce kindness.

To my big Italian and Portuguese families, thank you for the love, the big laughs, and the most amazing cheering section a girl could have. To the homestead Dolce Terra compound, you have made our quarantine pod an amazing blessing. I love each of you. I am so lucky to have married into the family.

To my Mom and Dad, who gave me everything and more than that. I love you with my whole heart and I count my blessings for you every day. To my brother Jeff and sister Dina, thanks for always being in my corner. I love you, sheesh.

To my boys, Giovanni, Casciato, and Roman, what joy and delight you bring! Thank you for your patience and shows of support during the many hours of me writing when you'd rather I'd be playing. It is an honor and privilege to be your mother.

To Rafael August, my husband, my best friend, my collaborator in all things. How I appreciate that we can share a profound soul experience, have a hip-hop dance-off while we clean the kitchen, and delight in the Warriors game, all in one day. I love you; my life truly began the day we found each other.

Finally, to the loving spirit that walks with me and guides me along. Thank you for the love and care that surrounds me. I hear and feel you everyday and I credit you for this book.

ABOUT THE AUTHOR

Melanie "Mel" Salvatore-August is a mama of three boys, veteran yoga/meditation teacher and teacher trainer, Reiki Master and author of *Fierce Kindness, Be a Positive Force For Change*; *Kitchen Yoga: Simple Home Practices to Transform Mind, Body & Life*, and now in 2021 release *Yoga to Support Immunity: A Mind Body Breathing Guide to Whole Health* (Mango Publishing).

Born in Pittsburgh, Pennsylvania, of Italian-American descent, her voice is warm, inclusive, practical, and filled with joy for life. With her early years as a classically trained actor, comedy/theatre writer-producer and as a teacher, she creates offerings that cultivate joy, personal growth, and freedom, elevating everyday challenges, humor, and spirit into one.

She is the founder of the Fierce Kindness Organization, and MELwell virtual studio. You can join Mel daily on the acclaimed YogaWorks-at-Home platform as well as her own MELwell studio.

Learn more at melaniesalvatoreaugust.com.

ABOUT THE ARTIST

Sebastian Alappat is a veteran art director and illustrator that left the corporate world to pursue his love for art. Following his heart led him to create SPARK, an art, yoga and meditation program serving children in New York City. Born in Kerala, India and immigrating to America at a young age, Sebastian grew up in Queens loving Batman, Spider-man and & the Mets. He lives in Harlem with his wife and two kids.

yellow pear 🍐 press

Yellow Pear Press, established in 2015, publishes inspiring, charming, clever, distinctive, playful, imaginative, beautifully designed lifestyle books, cookbooks, literary fiction, notecards, and journals with a certain *joie de vivre* in both content and style. Yellow Pear Press books have been honored by the Independent Publisher Book (IPPY) Awards, National Indie Excellence Awards, Independent Press Awards, and International Book Awards. Reviews of our titles have appeared in Kirkus Reviews, Foreword Reviews, Booklist, Midwest Book Review, San Francisco Chronicle, and New York Journal of Books, among others. Yellow Pear Press joined forces with Mango Publishing in 2020, both with the vision to continue publishing clever and innovative books. The fact that they're both named after fruit is a total coincidence.

We love hearing from our readers, so please stay in touch with us and follow us at:

- Facebook: Yellow Pear Press
- Instagram: @yellowpearpress
- Pinterest: yellowpearpress
- Website: www.mangopublishinggroup.com

9 781642 505726